30 MINUTES A DAY TO A HEALTHY HEART

One Simple Plan to Conquer All Six Major Threats to Your Heart

Frederic J. Vagnini, M.D., and Selene Yeager

Reader's Digest

The Reader's Digest Association, Inc.
Pleasantville, New York | Montreal

PROJECT STAFF

Contributing Writer
Sarí Harrar

Recipe Editor
Robyn Webb

Editor
Neil Wertheimer

Contributing Editor
Marianne Wait

Cover Designer
George McKeon

Book Designer
Rich Kershner

Illustrators
Shawn Banner (exercise)
Jess Koegel (decorative)
Marcia Hartsock (medical)

Copy Editor/Proofreaders
Jane Sherman
Jeanette Gingold

Indexer
Andrea Chesman

Managing Editor
Suzanne G. Beason

Art Director
Michele Laseau

Manufacturing Manager
John L. Cassidy

ISBN 13: 978-0-7621-0847-3
ISBN 10: 0-7621-0847-9

Reader's Digest Pocket Guide: 30 Minutes a Day to a Healthy Heart was previously published in a larger format as *30 Minutes a Day to a Healthy Heart* (ISBN: 0-7621-0678-6).

For more Reader's Digest products and information, visit our website:www.rd.com

NOTE TO OUR READERS

The information in this book should not be substituted for, or used to alter, medical therapy without your doctor's advice. For a specific health problem, consult your physician for guidance.

Printed in China

1   3   5   7   9   10   8   6   4   2

ABOUT THE AUTHORS

Frederic J. Vagnini, M.D., is a founder and head of the Cardiovascular Wellness Center in Long Island, New York. For 25 years he practiced as a heart, lung, and blood vessel surgeon. A frequent speaker and guest on local and national radio and TV, Dr. Vagnini also hosts a live weekly New York radio call-in show.

Selen Yeager is a top-selling professional health-and-fitness writer who lives what she writes as a certified personal trainer, triathlete, and mountain-bike racer. She has written, cowritten and contributed to more than a dozen books and is a contributing editor for *Prevention*, *Bicycling*, and *Scuba Diving*. Yeager lives in Emmaus, PA.

Robyn Webb (recipe editor) is founder and head of Pinch of Thyme, a healthy-cooking business that offers lessons, catering, and tours as well as providing nutritional counseling and consulting to corporations and government agencies.

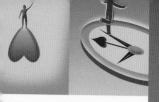

Contents

Introduction *4*

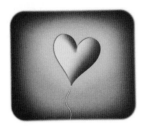

Introduction

HEART DISEASE HAS been America's top health problem for at least 100 years, and doctors have become amazingly smart on the topic. Today, we know what causes it, and we know how to treat it. We've created drugs that diminish its effects and developed advanced surgical procedures to mend the damage it causes. Given all that we know about heart disease, you'd think we'd be on the verge of eradicating it.

Sadly, nothing could be further from the truth. Heart disease is rampant in America and remains our top cause of death by far. And don't think for a moment that's mostly because of the aging of Americans: Heart-related diseases attack not only adults of *all* ages, but children as well.

Here's how sad the situation is. I was a heart, lung, and blood vessel surgeon for 25 years. During thousands of surgeries, I saw it all—damaged hearts barely able to beat, arteries with unimaginable disease inside, and atherosclerosis so bad that my best efforts failed to save lives.

Of all people, I should have known the importance of heart-healthy living, yet thanks to my own genetics—including a family history of obesity, heart disease, and diabetes—and my personal habits, my health started to deteriorate in my forties. I looked up one day to discover I was on the same path as my patients. I weighed over 300 pounds. My cholesterol was sky high, to the point that I had developed cholesterol deposits around my eyes. My liver was enlarged. I was short of breath and barely able to perform daily activities.

I wish I could say it was my career in heart surgery that caused me to turn my health around, but it was something more personal: having two small children. I knew I wouldn't be there for them if I didn't change course.

It was a long, difficult process, but today I'm strong, healthy, at a good weight, and thoroughly energized. I'm proud to say that my patients now say I'm a role model.

What did I do? Simple: I ate better. I started exercising. I took healthy supplements. I improved my attitude and managed my workload better. As a result, I not only got healthier, I looked and acted healthier, too. The changes, I'm told, were substantial.

The lesson? It's that for all the advances we've made in medical science, the real answer to heart disease lies in the art of living. I can say with complete certainty that all those drug therapies, surgical interventions, and other consequences of cardiovascular disease are preventable through lifestyle changes. Research shows it, and so does the success of thousands of my own patients and millions of other people who have chosen healthy living.

Despite this, heart disease, obesity, diabetes, and stroke still plague us. Why? When I stopped doing heart surgery and turned my efforts to clinical nutrition and preventive medicine, I found that most heart patients didn't know how to improve their diets or fitness levels. The medical field is at least partly to blame because it isn't equipped to offer counseling, prevention, and risk reduction. There's no time and no financial reimbursement for them. Physicians today are too busy caring for the sick to have time for the healthy.

My personal goal is more prevention. I see daily in my practice that the right diet, exercise, stress reduction measures, and nutritional counseling lead to unbelievable improvement in health, well-being, and longevity. I know that when people start to use the principles of healthy living, they will experience an unbelievable "body makeover" and a huge drop in heart disease risk.

This book provides those principles in a health plan based on the best science around, as well as on the success of thousands of patients. Here are also several breakthrough ideas about heart health, things you haven't read anywhere else. We've worked hard to make this book as fresh, contemporary, and useful as possible.

For example, we've coined a new term: sitting disease. Can you believe that many of us sit or lie around for as many as 23 hours a day? Sedentary living is one of the biggest risk factors for heart disease, but moving more is simple and delivers amazing heart benefits!

We're also among the first to say to a broad audience that all of the major risk factors for heart disease—including obesity, high blood pressure, high cholesterol, and chronic inflammation—are interconnected. This, too, is a breakthrough idea. For too long, we've been fixated on blood

> For all the advances in medical science, the real answer to heart disease lies in the art of living.

pressure readings or cholesterol counts without putting them in the broader context of heart health and long life. Yes, these are important components of arterial health, but they shouldn't be treated in isolation. They're intertwined, as are several other conditions that affect the heart.

For this reason, we've focused the advice in this book on lifestyle changes that science shows can reduce the risk of each of the major heart attackers—hence our claim that one plan can conquer all major heart threats. It's a bold assertion but absolutely true, based on research and extensive clinical experience.

We also claim fast results. Again, both experience and research confirm it. Studies show that healthy eating, exercise, stress reduction, and certain supplements can have a measurable effect on arterial health within 24 hours. Studies on smoking cessation also show that lung function can improve in less than 48 hours after quitting.

There are many books about heart health, but after I attended the first editorial meeting for 30 Minutes a Day to a Healthy Heart, I knew immediately that we had something new and better to say, and the right team to say it. We were impassioned, and that passion has been successfully transferred to these pages. As I say each week on my radio show, your health is in your hands. Today, I mean that literally. The book you are holding truly provides the antidote to heart disease. Read it and take action for a longer, stronger, and happier life.

FREDERIC J. VAGNINI, M.D., F.A.C.S.

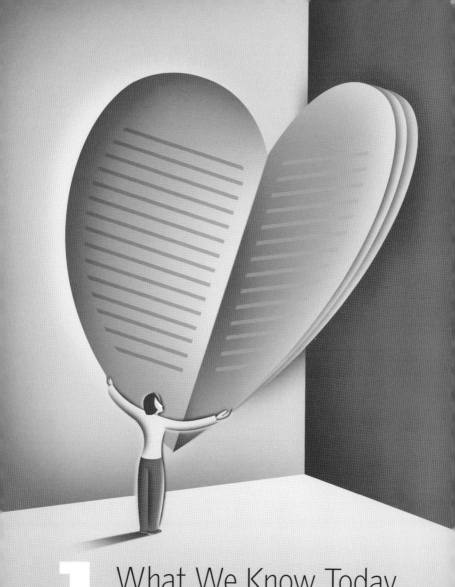

1 What We Know Today About Your Heart

The human heart, when well nourished and cherished, will provide you a surprising abundance of energized, happy years.

Your Heart's Full Potential

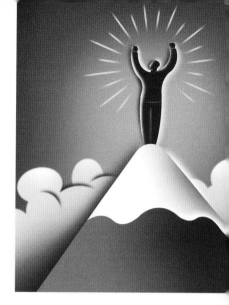

IN A PERFECT WORLD, your heart would *not* stop—suddenly, unexpectedly, painfully—at age 45, 55, or 65, as the hearts of a half million American women and men do each year. It would pump bravely and joyfully on, breezing by seemingly impossible odds to survive well past your 100th birthday.

High-tech clinical experiments and investigations of the world's oldest living people concur on this exciting point: Your heart *wasn't* built to give out in the prime of life. It was built to last—possibly, longevity experts speculate, until you've reached the ripe, very old age of 120. Yet too often, this ingenious, fist-size pump—a glorious, always-beating machine made of muscle, nerves, arteries, and electrical transmitters—is done in by everyday temptations (the triple cheeseburger! The *Survivor*

reruns!) and a modern world that zips along faster than we ever thought possible.

Living proof of your heart's untapped potential? Consider the residents of Okinawa, a Japanese island-state in the East China Sea that's home to the world's highest proportion of folks over the age of 100. Okinawa has 35 centenarians for every 100,000 residents; America has 10. Thanks to a traditional lifestyle that prizes serenity and spirituality; daily exercise; and a low-calorie diet that's light on saturated fat and heavy on fruit, vegetables, soy, and fish, Okinawa's death rates from coronary heart disease are *82 percent* lower than U.S. rates.

Carved into a stone marker facing the sea in one tiny Okinawan fishing village is this ancient local saying:

At 70, you are still a child, at 80, a young man or woman. And if at 90, someone from

Heaven invites you over, tell him: "Just go away, and come back when I am 100!"

Living Health

Western journalists flocked to Okinawa after researchers brought its super-heart-healthy lifestyle to world attention. What they found: Vibrant lives, well lived—without drugs, nursing homes, or life-support systems. A 100-year-old villager outdrank a TV film crew half her age. A 96-year-old martial artist trounced a 30-ish boxing champion on national television. A 105-year-old woman became a neighborhood legend when she killed a poisonous snake with her flyswatter.

Meanwhile, medical tests revealed why these feats were possible: The centenarians had remarkably healthy hearts, young-looking arteries, low cholesterol, and little of the oxidative stress that spurs atherosclerosis, the dangerous plaque buildup that spawns heart-stopping blood clots.

Even more surprising: Researchers who have studied 600 of Okinawa's oldest residents conclude that healthy lifestyle accounts for 80 percent of the super health enjoyed by their hearts, and genetics is responsible for a mere 20 percent. What's more, they say, if Americans lived more like these folks, one in five U.S. coronary care units could be permanently shut down. Of course, to get there, we'd have to learn the art of living Okinawa-style—including a slow, lower-calorie eating practice called *hara hachi bu*, which means eating until you're just 80 percent full; a relaxed outlook on life called *taygay*; and deep, meditative spirituality.

Heart Disease Around the World

Death rates from cardiovascular disease—the clogged arteries that can cause heart attacks and brain-damaging strokes—vary widely from nation to nation, a reflection of global differences in diet and lifestyle. Here's the lowdown—the number of deaths per year linked to cardiovascular disease per 100,000 people.

Russia	945
Romania	817
Poland	669
Scotland	432
Finland	416
United States	348
Germany	347
England	332
Canada	280
China	266
Korea	261
Switzerland	249
Australia	237
Brazil	230
India	225
France	206
Japan	186

The past few decades have brought sad proof that Okinawan heart health is not the result of lucky genes; island residents under age 50 now have the highest heart disease rates in Japan, thanks to Westernized diets and lifestyles.

This real-world lesson in the care and feeding of the human heart is echoed in findings from population studies around the world. Greenland's native Inuit people have dramatically lower rates of heart disease than the Danish neighbors who share their icy little continent, thanks to a diet rich in fish loaded with heart-nurturing omega-3 fatty acids, notes the Icelandic Longevity Institute. Researchers from the Harvard School of Public Health found that Greeks who stuck with the traditional Mediterranean diet—brimming with sun-ripened produce, beans, local olive oil, and, you guessed it, fish, had at least a 25 percent lower risk of heart disease than those who did not. And in the United States, a study of New Englanders who've passed the 100-year milestone found that while diet matters, living a fully heart-smart life is what really counts. These American centenarians were lean, fit nonsmokers—and they had personalities and coping skills that equipped them to handle stress well.

It takes a whole person, living a fully healthy life, to nurture a healthy heart. When researchers at the University of Pittsburgh Medical Center attempted to keep a human heart alive by artificial means outside the body, it stopped beating in 12 hours. Clearly, your heart works best in the company of a sound body and a happy mind.

Heart Disease in America

Ah, but welcome to the modern life— where modern hearts are in grave and constant peril despite 30 years of revolutionary advances in every aspect of cardiology, the science of heart health and disease. Doctors know precisely which chemical cocktails will keep your cholesterol low and your blood pressure calm; biologists can describe—molecule by molecule—the biochemical drama that pumps plaque into artery walls like so much custard into a greasy doughnut; geneticists can pinpoint exactly which bits of the human genome are responsible for heightened heart attack risk; and it seems that every week, a hot new heart risk is discovered—and a remedy found. Yet this year alone, 1.5 million Americans will have heart attacks. Up to one-third will die from them.

Nothing kills more American women and men, whether in old age or the prime of life, than cardiovascular disease. Add together the deaths caused by the nation's other top five killers— cancer, accidents, respiratory disease, diabetes, and strokes—and you still won't equal the heart disease body count.

Nothing disables more Americans, either. Among the survivors of heart attacks, one in five men and nearly one in two women live the rest of their lives with the disabling fatigue and worry of heart failure—heart-muscle death that happens after a clot chokes off the blood supply during a heart attack. Many ultimately need heart transplants and will die waiting for them, and *all* survivors live with the big fear that the next one's just around the corner. Within six years of their first heart attacks, 18 percent of male survivors and 35 percent of female survivors will have second attacks.

How could this be happening in 21st-century America? The truth is, we know more *facts* about the human heart than ever

It takes a whole person, living a fully healthy life, to nurture a healthy heart.

before, yet we treat our own tickers with little respect and less understanding. We live in a world that threatens our hearts like never before. We eat too much and move too little. As a result, most of us are overweight or downright obese. Our food choices are stunningly *un*healthy, and they flood our bodies with the worst types of fats and carbohydrates while starving it of the good fats, fiber, and antioxidants that "feed" longevity. What's more, we live in states of intense stress that boosts levels of damaging stress hormones and leaves us little time for the heart-nurturing company of our family and friends and comforting spirituality.

The vulnerable, ever-beating pump that keeps us alive wasn't built for the onslaughts of the 21st century. In order to work 24/7, the heart muscle demands a constant supply of oxygen-rich blood, delivered via a network of coronary arteries. If these thread-thin arteries become constricted by plaque or blocked by a clot, the heart faces an immediate oxygen deficit. It's a deadly crisis. Oxygen-starved heart muscle

hurts—that's the short-lived chest pain called angina. Worse, oxygen-deprived heart muscle can die quickly, leading to heart failure, heart attack, and even death.

Women's Hearts Break, Too

If you think heart disease is strictly a man's problem, consider this: One in every two American women will die of heart disease. That's a staggering 248,000 deaths this year alone, more than all female deaths from stroke and cancer combined.

Even more shocking: Most women are more worried about breast cancer, and many doctors, who as late as the 1980s didn't even believe that women developed heart disease, still overlook uniquely female cardiovascular risks, even to the point of misdiagnosing and dismissing women's heart attacks *while they're happening*.

What's going on? According to Nancy Loving, who survived a heart attack in her forties and is a cofounder of the National Coalition for Women with Heart Disease,

Is It a Heart Attack? Call 911

Think you may be having a heart attack? Don't mull it over—call 911 and let the experts decide. Most heart attack deaths happen in the first hour after an attack begins, yet many people wait *several hours* before calling for help. If you or someone you love has chest pain or any of the telltale symptoms listed here for

more than a few minutes, call an ambulance immediately.

Chest discomfort. Most heart attacks involve discomfort in the center of the chest that lasts more than a few minutes or goes away and comes back. It can be uncomfortable pressure, squeezing, fullness, or pain.

Discomfort in other areas of the upper body. Symptoms

can include pain or discomfort in one or both arms, the back, neck, jaw, or stomach.

Shortness of breath. This symptom may occur with or without chest discomfort.

Other signs. These may include breaking out in a cold sweat, nausea, lightheadedness, or overwhelming fatigue.

women's hearts are held hostage by two myths: *Only men have heart disease,* and *women are at risk only in old age.* The truth is that eight million American women are living with heart disease—that's 10 percent of all women between the ages of 45 and 64 and 25 percent of those 65 and older. More than 435,000 women have heart attacks each year—and more than half die. In fact, while heart attack rates for men are falling, rates for women are on the rise.

Overlooked? You bet. Women comprise only 25 percent of participants in all heart-related research studies, leaving family docs without the data they need to recognize and treat women. The result? "In my whole life, not one doctor spoke to me about heart disease, even though they knew my father and three uncles died young of heart attacks. Then, bingo—I have a heart attack at age 48. I guess they figured heart disease was a guy thing," says one member of the coalition.

Here's what you need to know.

- **Women downplay their own risks.** In a recent survey, one-half of all U.S. women knew heart disease was a major health issue, yet just 13 percent considered it a *personal* health concern.

- **Many women's heart attacks don't include classic chest pain.** A new study of more than 500 female heart attack survivors found that top symptoms were shortness of breath, feeling weak and/or fatigued, breaking into a cold sweat, and dizziness—not the classic heart attack signs recognized by most emergency medical personnel. Forty-three percent felt no chest pain at all.

Feel the Beat

Your heart rate—the number of beats per minute—can help you and your doctor assess your heart's fitness. A normal range is 60 to 80 beats per minute while you're resting. A faster beat may simply indicate that you just ran up the stairs so you wouldn't be late for your doctor's appointment (physical activity boosts heart rate). Fever; a short illness such as a cold, the flu, or a stomach bug; and anxiety can also cause a temporary elevation. But a consistently fast resting heartbeat can be a sign of trouble, such as anemia, thyroid problems, or a cardiovascular defect.

To check your heart rate, make sure you have been resting for 5 to 10 minutes. Have a clock or watch with a second hand ready, then use the pads of your fingers to find your pulse—try your inner wrist or your neck. Count the beats for 6 seconds, then multiply by 10.

- **38 percent of women will die within one year of a first heart attack, compared to 25 percent of men.** Yet women receive less treatment and get less medication (such as beta blockers, ACE inhibitors, and even aspirin) after heart attacks. They also receive only about one-third of all procedures to open blocked arteries.

- **Menopause is a defining moment for women and heart disease.** Before menopause, a woman's naturally high estrogen levels protect her heart. After menopause, women have higher cholesterol levels, which may raise the risk of heart disease, especially in the presence of high triglycerides, a powerful contributor to heart disease. In general, women with high triglycerides (over 150 mg/dl) and low HDL (under 50 mg/dl) have greater risks for heart disease than do men with similar levels.

- **The causes of heart disease are different for women.** For example, type 2 diabetes boosts heart disease risk more in women than in men. Women who smoke are twice as likely to have heart attacks as male smokers. Depression is also a stronger heart risk factor for women than for men.

- **Women have risk factors that men don't face.** Taking birth control pills is one example: High blood pressure is two to three times more common in women who take oral contraceptives—especially in those who are overweight. Also, women whose blood pressure rises during pregnancy, then returns to normal after delivery, are more likely to have high blood pressure later in life.

What about hormone replacement therapy (HRT)? Until just a few years ago, doctors recommended HRT to post-menopausal women as a heart protector. In 2002, the government's landmark Women's Health Initiative (WHI) found it didn't shield hearts at all and in fact raised the risk of blood clots in the first year or so. "Hormone therapy should not be used to prevent cardiovascular disease," says JoAnn Manson, M.D., chief of preventive medicine at Brigham and Women's Hospital in Boston and one of the WHI's lead investigators.

What every woman should do: Understand your personal heart risk, then eat smart, move around, de-stress, track your crucial heart health numbers (including weight, waist measurement, cholesterol, and blood pressure), and keep your doctor updated on your progress.

It's good advice for men, too. So why do we all keep missing this simple truth?

Shift Your Focus

Your life depends on the health of your coronary arteries, but these key blood vessels are no match for the fat in a stuffed-crust pizza; endless sitting in cars, behind desks, and glued to 500-channel cable TV; or the stress of 60-hour workweeks. Nor can they battle the cumulative impact of dozens of little "should haves," such as the dental floss gathering dust in your medicine cabinet, the exercise-bike-turned-clothes-tree in your laundry room, the old friends you haven't had time to see lately, and the yoga video you keep meaning to watch again but never quite get around to.

Instead of living powerfully heart-smart lives, we focus on the wrong things, hoping the latest scientific developments will rescue our ailing tickers. Newspapers and TV news channels trumpet each new heart study that bursts from a lab. Likewise, they jump on incremental scientific findings as the next breakthrough that will solve all our heart problems. Not having degrees in medicine, we listen—and believe.

What causes heart attacks? Doctors can describe the process in horrific medical detail—and all too often, they do. It is arterial plaque and hardening of the arteries. It's damage to your arteries caused by free radicals and excessive blood pressure. It's chronic inflammation within your body and the bad body chemistry it creates. It's a host of fats, oils, hormones, and other body chemicals in your bloodstream that shouldn't be there.

All that is true from a narrow, scientific perspective. But what really causes heart disease is much simpler: It's how we live.

In late 2004, a major study involving 30,000 people across the globe showed that 90 percent of heart attacks were caused by just nine risk factors. Five of them were purely lifestyle choices: smoking, stress, sedentary living, eating too few fruits and vegetables, and perhaps most surprising, abstaining from alcohol! (Later, we'll explain why having one or two drinks a day is so healthy for you.)

The remaining four are more medical in nature, but don't be fooled—each one is closely and directly linked to lifestyle choices. The four are abnormal cholesterol levels, diabetes, high blood pressure, and abdominal obesity.

What's intriguing and important about this study is that it spanned 52 countries and involved men and women of all ages, races, and socioeconomic backgrounds. It revealed that whether you are a poor woman in Chicago or a rich man in Tokyo, the exact same risk factors cause heart attacks—mostly sitting too much, eating poorly, and being overly stressed.

So don't be one of those people who are waiting for science to protect their hearts. The truth is—and it's one of the most important truths in this book—that a healthy lifestyle can vanquish all the medical causes of heart attacks *at the same time*.

Yes, it is good to know what the various threats are, and we give you a concise, well-informed roundup of the six major ones in the next chapter. Our real goal with this book, however, is to show you how to take them *all* on with one simple program that goes after their root cause—our sedentary, calorie-and-fat-laden, TV-watching, stressed-out modern lives.

Animals *Do* Get Heart Disease

News flash from the animal kingdom: Pigs die of heart attacks. Pigeons, parrots, rabbits, and wild howler monkeys develop atherosclerosis. So do the wild turkeys that roam America's woodlands—in fact, those from Michigan seem to have the most artery-choking plaque, and those in Indiana have the least, reports the *American Journal of Veterinary Research*. And baboons?

Despite their strict vegetarian diet and active lifestyle, many have mildly elevated cholesterol.

So much for the theory—or myth—that animals are free of heart disease. The truth is far more interesting: Plant-munching herbivores are as vulnerable to atherosclerosis as humans are. In contrast, 100 percent meat eaters seem to have arteries lined with Teflon: Lions, tigers, housecats,

pet dogs (except Dobermans), and other carnivores simply don't get atherosclerosis, even if they're force-fed saturated fat and cholesterol. Why? Carnivores convert most of the fat they eat into heart-protecting HDL cholesterol, while the bodies of herbivores and omnivores (such as humans, who eat plants and meat) convert more dietary fat into artery-choking LDL cholesterol.

The Path to a Healthy Heart

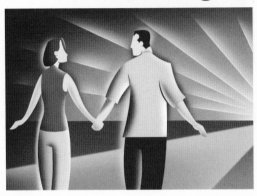

This is the foundation of the 30-Minutes-A-Day Plan. We've found the simplest, most powerful steps you can take—without adding more jobs to your to-do list or expenses to your monthly budget—to protect your heart the way nature intended.

Heart-smart living can be as simple as laughing at a bad situation rather than getting angry. It means going for walks after dinner, not watching game shows or sports. It means having an apple for dessert rather than apple pie, or spending 15 minutes sipping a cup of homemade cocoa (check our extra-healthy recipe on page 102) curled up on the sofa with your spouse instead of watching the 11 o'clock news with a bag of chips. It's doing a 5-minutes-a-day strength-training program while the coffee perks in the morning or taking a 3-second meditative pause when the "you've got mail" alert sounds on your computer.

Our message: At a cost of no more than 30 minutes a day, you can take powerful, scientifically proven steps to overcome the biggest heart threats out there, including tummy fat, high cholesterol, high blood pressure, insulin resistance, inflammation, free radicals, and a host of factors researchers are still striving to understand, such as homocysteine and a cholesterol particle called LP(a).

Here's the plan (the rest of this book will give you the details) that lets you take them all on and win.

1. FOCUS ON SMALL CHANGES FOR BIG RESULTS

Fast, simple diet swaps can cut cholesterol by 30 percent. A 5-minutes-a-day weight-training program can replace 10 years' worth of lost muscle tissue. This book is packed with timesaving lifestyle changes that get results, don't cost a fortune, and are easy to stick with for the long haul.

2. CONQUER SITTING DISEASE

Americans spend 22 hours a day sitting or lying down, yet our bodies are built for lots and lots of daily activity. We'll show you how to build healthy movement back into your life, no matter how jam-packed your days are.

3. EAT FRESH FOODS

Fresh, whole foods don't have to cost more or take more time to prepare than the packaged stuff. These wholesome, delicious edibles—fresh fruits and veggies, grains, fish, meats, dairy products, and even soy—not only taste good, they also protect your heart by slashing blood fats, driving down elevated blood sugar, cooling off inflammation, and fighting destructive free radicals. We'll show you the easiest way to start eating healthier foods and fewer foods from a box.

4. KNOW YOUR NUMBERS

You want results? You can track your success by keeping tabs on six crucial numbers. All adult Americans should know where they stand with regard to these numbers, but virtually none do. You may be surprised by the list, both what's on it and what's not. For help sticking with the program, we'll also tell you which four things to monitor on a daily basis—a task that should take about 30 seconds each evening. It's that simple.

The Heart Attackers

Doctors vigorously debate this list, but based on our best current knowledge, here are the primary medical conditions that affect the heart and that the health industry is most focused on understanding and curing, along with the page on which we give a full briefing.

The Six Major Attackers

Additional Attackers

---

5. AVOID TOXINS

From tobacco to trans fats, sugar to environmental pollutants, the "toxins" we allow to enter our bodies seem to wreak havoc with our hearts first. Your body doesn't have to be a Superfund site. We'll show you how to clean it up.

6. FIND JOY

A growing stack of research links hostility, impatience, and holding grudges with poor heart health; in contrast, forgiveness, friends, and optimism are linked with healthier hearts. Do you have a heart-threatening personality type? Find out—and learn how to live a more joyful life.

Follow our 30-Minutes-A-Day Plan, and the chances are huge that you will successfully defeat not just one or two of the heart attackers but all of them. As a side benefit, you'll have greater energy, a happier attitude, a more attractive body, and fewer minor health problems such as colds and digestive troubles. Aren't a few well-spent minutes a day a small amount to ask for such amazing benefits?

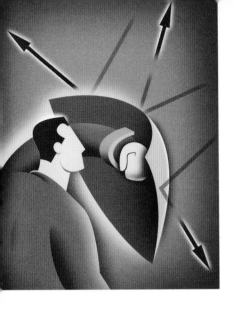

The 6 Deadly Heart Attackers

EACH MONTH, MAJOR medical journals publish hundreds of studies about heart disease, covering everything from A (for artery-clearing angioplasty) to X (for xanthoma, a cholesterol deposit under the skin). The National Library of Medicine, which maintains the world's most comprehensive database of published health research, lists more than 500,000 research papers about heart disease alone!

Despite all that knowledge, a half million Americans die from heart disease each year, while researchers work to reveal the heart's inner workings in ever more exquisite detail. In a sense, the details are deadly.

Here's why. The nature of medical research is to focus on very narrow questions—for example, whether an increase in intake of a particular nutrient causes any change in a particular body chemical. The

age-old "forest for the trees" expression applies well here: If the proverbial forest is the human heart, and each tree in the forest is one aspect of what affects the heart (cholesterol, vitamins, exercise, and so on), then the typical medical study focuses on a single branch of a tree. What emerges, then, is an overwhelming number of studies focusing on small details that by themselves reveal very little about the big picture. Very few doctors—and even fewer health journalists—have had the time or wisdom to synthesize all the research into a unified view of total heart health.

That affects us. We get all caught up with single issues, such as high cholesterol or high blood pressure, when each is just one tree—albeit a major one—in the forest.

The truth is, major heart risks are interwoven—they rarely occur individually.

Researchers and drug companies are beginning to catch on to this heart truth: In a study published in the journal *Archives of Internal Medicine*, Mayo Clinic researchers discovered that among 2,300 people with known high blood pressure, two-thirds also had high cholesterol and/or high triglycerides, yet for 9 out of 10, these other heart risks went untreated. And early in 2004, the FDA approved the first combination drug to treat high blood pressure and high cholesterol. "The two conditions are intrinsically linked," notes Craig Hopkinson, M.D., medical director of the drug's manufacturer, Pfizer Cardiovascular. In fact, 55 percent of people diagnosed with high blood pressure also have high cholesterol, and 43 percent of people diagnosed with high cholesterol also have high blood pressure—whether they know it or not.

Isn't it time you looked beyond the details, too? That's what the 30-Minutes-A-Day Plan is all about: Showing you the big picture—plus giving you a plan that wallops all the attackers at once. When you treat yourself as one gloriously integrated system—mind, body, and spirit—achieving heart health is so much easier. The bonus? You'll also cut your risk of diabetes, cancer, and other major health conditions.

Lurking: The Attackers

You may wonder why, if one plan can reduce all of the major risks to your heart, you should bother learning about each one. There are a few answers. First, the media talks an awful lot about these risks—often mistakenly. Learning the truth will give you the knowledge to help put the "news" in perspective and keep you focused on what matters. Even more, knowing how the heart attackers interconnect, and how certain lifestyle choices can affect several at once, is very empowering. You'll be far more convinced of the power of the 30-Minutes-A-Day Plan when you understand its basis.

Major heart risks are interwoven— they rarely occur singly.

So, here's what you need to know: A concise briefing on the six most troublesome attackers that your heart faces. In the next 30 minutes of reading (consider it today's installment of the 30-Minutes-A-Day Plan!), you'll become an instant expert on the heart topics that matter most.

You'll see how conventional wisdom about heart disease has evolved over the past 50 years—from a simplistic view of health to today's sophisticated view. You'll discover how each attacker develops in your body, trace the ways our 21st-century lifestyles fuel these menaces, and learn how to assess your risk for each. You'll also see the strong links among the six major attackers: for example, how belly fat fuels at least three other attackers and how sitting disease—21st-century super-sedentary living—powers high blood pressure, oxidative stress, and all the rest.

Are you ready for some important and empowering knowledge? Grab a cup of tea and read on.

Excess Body Fat

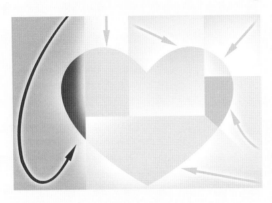

Once, fat was America's ultimate status symbol—a sign of health and wealth, sex appeal and fertility, all rolled into one plump bundle. Before the dawn of the 20th century, a skinny physique indicated a personal history of sickness, meager meals, and little money. Even in life insurance circles, fat was considered a smart hedge against disease.

That was then, this is now—the era of Krispy Kremes and Big Gulps, and desk-jockey days followed by TV-and-Internet nights. Today, excess body fat is the status quo: 64 percent of Americans—including nearly 30 million adults—are overweight.

What's more, the obesity epidemic is deadly serious. In 2000, according to astonishing study results published by the Centers for Disease Control and Prevention (CDC), obesity caused 400,000 deaths in the United States, compared with 435,000 deaths from smoking. "If this trend continues, it will soon overtake tobacco," says CDC director Julie L. Gerberding, M.D. Her agency predicts that soon it will be the nation's number one killer.

How can love handles and a potbelly be so deadly? A growing stack of research reveals that killer fat is *visceral fat*—the stuff packed around (and sometimes *in*) your internal organs. While hip, thigh, and butt fat are relatively benign, belly fat ratchets up your odds for high blood pressure, blood clots, and cholesterol trouble. Belly fat also starts a chain of biochemical events that leads to insulin resistance—a precursor of type 2 diabetes, heart disease, stroke, breast and prostate cancer, and even kidney failure and Alzheimer's disease.

Why? The conventional view of fat cells—as safe-deposit boxes shut tightly until your body needs extra energy—doesn't apply to visceral fat. It's *active* fat, which continually pumps into your bloodstream artery-clogging fatty acids that your liver converts into "bad guy" LDL cholesterol. Visceral fat also releases other compounds—among them, appetite-regulating hormones and immune system chemicals—that open the door for three huge heart risks: atherosclerosis, metabolic syndrome, and inflammation. "We believe that this hidden fat is the most dangerous fat in the body," says Osama Hamdy, M.D., director of the obesity clinic at the Joslin Diabetes Center in Boston.

Top-heavy women and men—nicknamed "apples"—carry more central fat, even if they're slim everyplace else, while "pears," whose weight collects on their hips and thighs, have less. When is a thick waist risky? Grab a tape measure and wrap it snugly around the narrowest part of your naked waist (*don't* suck in your belly). Generally, men with waists over 40 inches and women with waists over 35 inches are at higher risk. We consider visceral fat so serious that we've named waist measurement as one of the six most important numbers to track for your health (for more details, see "6 Numbers That Can Save Your Life" on page 207).

How can you get rid of this fat? In the future, surgeons may simply pull it out. Obesity experts recently completed a stunning bit of experimental fat-reduction surgery, removing strips of yellow-hued visceral fat through tiny incisions in the abdomens of four obese volunteers. The study participants' body chemistry improved almost immediately.

Don't wait for surgery, though; you can trim this vicious stuff now. How? On the 30-Minutes-A-Day-Plan, you'll eat less saturated fat and virtually no trans fats, because diets high in "sat fats"—such as butter, fatty meats, ice cream, and full-fat milk—pack on the central fat, as do trans fats, which give many commercial cookies, crackers, and chips their crunch. You'll up your fiber intake—a move proven in a Harvard study to visibly whittle visceral fat. You'll relax and enjoy life, because daily stress and high levels of the stress hormone cortisol are intimately linked with visceral fat storage. And, you'll be moving. In an eight-month study of 170 overweight people at Duke University Medical Center, those who exercised vigorously cut visceral fat by 8 percent, while sedentary folks accumulated 5 to 11 percent more of it.

WHAT'S YOUR RISK?

Excess Body Fat

Is your weight in the danger zone? One of the most popular measures today is BMI, or body mass index, which takes into account both weight and height. Many Web sites and health reference books have large tables that help you find your number, but if you have a calculator, here's how to determine your precise BMI. It's a good number to know, since most doctors, other health experts, and insurers use it to gauge the healthiness of your weight.

1. Multiply your weight in pounds by 703.
2. Divide the answer by your height in inches.
3. Divide that answer by your height in inches.

For example, if you're 5 feet 5 inches tall (that's 65 inches) and weigh 140 pounds, your BMI is 23.3:

1. $140 \times 703 = 98,420$
2. $98,420 \div 65 = 1514.2$
3. $1514.2 \div 65 = 23.3$

For adults ages 20 and older, BMI rankings fall into the following categories.

BMI	RANKING
18.5 and below	Underweight
18.6 to 24.9	Normal
25 to 29.9	Overweight
30 and above	Obese

#1 BODY FAT: WHAT YOU NEED TO KNOW

Your body naturally contains millions of fat cells. Each one is an expandable pouch filled with fat droplets, called lipids, that are made of fats, sugars, and amino acids derived from the foods you eat. Under normal circumstances, your body uses fat tissue to cushion bones, to regulate temperature, and as fuel when blood sugar runs low.

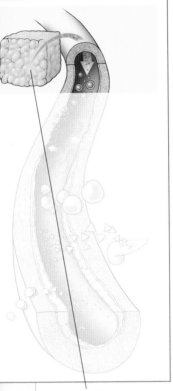

Abdominal fat continually pumps fatty acids and chemicals into the bloodstream that can lead to atherosclerosis, chronic inflammation, and metabolic syndrome.

HOW IT ACCUMULATES: When you eat more food than your body needs to function, fat cells expand until they fill to capacity. If there is still an abundance of calories to be stored, your body manufactures new fat cells. (Until recently, experts believed the human body stopped producing new fat cells after puberty. Now they know that overeating can trigger fat cell production in adults.)

WHAT'S NEW:

Visceral fat. Not all body fat is equally bad. The body's most dangerous fat collects in your abdominal cavity, nestling around internal organs. This visceral fat pumps out hormones that upset body chemistry, significantly upping your risk of heart disease and other major conditions.

The role of carbohydrates. Research is confirming that eating an excessive amount of simple carbohydrates (i.e., sugar, white flour, rice, potatoes) contributes to weight gain, lending credence to a core principle of the low-carb weight-loss movement.

DETECTING IT: That's easy: Look in the mirror. Check your BMI. Step on a scale. Measure your waist. Overweight is the easiest health condition to measure and monitor.

STANDARD MEDICAL CARE: We spend $39 billion a year on prescription diet drugs, weight-loss surgery, diet programs, over-the-counter weight-loss supplements, health clubs, diet sodas, and artificial sweeteners. Buyer beware: Most claims for over-the-counter weight-loss pills are overstated. Prescription drugs, which typically suppress appetite or block fat absorption, usually produce only modest weight loss, and weight-loss surgery is sometimes risky.

Researchers are testing the potential of several hormones to curb appetite. They're also looking at ways to subdue ghrelin, the so-called hunger hormone. So far, none of this research has resulted in a commercially available weight-loss drug.

VIABILITY OF SELF-TREATMENT: Very high for most people. Healthy eating, physical activity, and improved stress management will reduce body fat over time in most cases.

Cholesterol

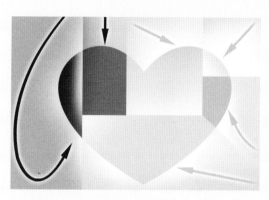

Cholesterol burst on the scene in the 1950s, grabbing headlines and giving America a grim new heart attack equation—too much saturated fat in the diet equals too much cholesterol in the bloodstream equals clogged arteries and heart attacks. Despite the fact that heart disease has been the nation's leading cause of death since 1921, nobody wanted to hear that the good things in life—butter, cheese, ice cream, and fat-marbled steaks sizzling on grills on thousands of suburban patios—just might spell doom.

The story centers on University of Minnesota researcher Ancel Keys, Ph.D.

During World War II, Dr. Keys developed the infamous K rations that fueled the American military. In the early 1950s, he noticed that well-nourished American businessmen had soaring rates of heart disease, while rates among people living through food shortages in postwar Europe declined.

The connection was startling (and aspects of Dr. Keys's research is often criticized today). After studying men in seven countries—Finland, Greece, Yugoslavia, Italy, the Netherlands, Japan, and the United States—and comparing their blood cholesterol levels, intake of saturated fats, and cardiovascular disease rates, Dr. Keys concluded that a "strong association" existed between saturated fats and heart health. One 1950s pop-culture Web site calls it "the day the pork rinds died."

Dr. Keys, who made the cover of *Time* magazine, recommended cutting saturated fat and eating more polyunsaturated fats (such as corn oil) to lower total cholesterol levels. Less total cholesterol, he reasoned, would lead to fewer heart attack deaths. It was the basis for America's first heart-healthy "prudent diet," recommended by the newly formed American Heart Association in 1957.

But, as it turned out, the cholesterol story wasn't that simple.

Fast-forward to the 21st century. Cholesterol isn't necessarily a villain. Your liver (and your intestines and even your skin) manufactures this soft, waxy stuff every day to help your body build cell membranes and produce sex hormones, vitamin D, and fat-digesting bile acids. The raw material for your body's cholesterol? The fat in your diet.

The real key to heart-healthy cholesterol levels, experts now say, isn't simply getting a lower total cholesterol number on a blood test. It's a smart balance between two basic types: "bad," low-density, lipoproteins (LDLs) and "good," high-density, lipoproteins (HDLs). The latest news: Heart experts are finding that the higher your HDLs and the lower your LDLs—essentially, the closer you can come to the "natural" cholesterol balance discovered in hunter-gatherer societies—the lower your risk for clogged coronary arteries and heart attack.

LDLs: The Lower, the Better

Like Federal Express trucks packed with fat droplets, LDLs are designed to efficiently navigate the bloodstream, delivering liquefied cholesterol directly to your cells. The problem comes when too many LDLs crowd the blood, then burrow into the tissue-thin inner lining of arteries, forming the foundation for heart-threat-

Cholesterol

As you've learned, one type of cholesterol—called LDL—is bad for you, and so you want as low a reading as possible for that type, preferably under 100 milligrams per deciliter of blood. The other cholesterol—HDL—is good for you, and so you want a reading above 60 mg/dl. Together, you want them to add up to below 200.

LDL (mg/dl)	RISK
Under 100	Optimal
100–129	Near optimal
130–159	Borderline high
160–189	High
190 and above	Very high

HDL (mg/dl)	BENEFIT
Under 40	Low
40-59	Average
60 and above	High

ening plaques in artery walls. Over time, these plaques—a mix of fat, cholesterol, calcium, and other cellular sludge—can narrow coronary arteries so less blood flows to your heart muscle. New research also suggests that one type of LDLs—small, dense LDLs—is particularly lethal. These tightly packed particles are easily damaged by free radicals in the bloodstream and then enter artery walls with ease, setting the scene for the plaque buildup of atherosclerosis. (For more on small, dense LDLs, read about oxidative stress on page 38).

The bottom line? High amounts of LDLs in your bloodstream up your risk of atherosclerosis. Low levels reduce your risk: For every one-point drop in LDLs, heart risk falls by 2 percent. LDLs and HDLs are measured according to their amounts per

volume of blood, expressed in milligrams per deciliter, or mg/dl.

Where's the safety zone? All research indicates that you should shoot for a two-digit LDL number, meaning under 100 mg/dl. In a provocative study published in March 2004 in the *Journal of the American Medical Association,* researchers from the Cleveland Clinic found that high doses of cholesterol-lowering medications to push LDL levels below 100 mg/dl halted the progression of heart disease and cut mortality rates by 28 percent. "We stopped heart disease in its tracks," says lead researcher Steven Nissen, M.D. "This shook up the lipid world."

While Dr. Nissen's results were achieved with statin drugs, the 30-Minutes-A-Day Plan could help you cut your LDLs by 30 percent. How?

You'll cut saturated fat, conquer sitting disease, and control a range of newly discovered heart risks—such as chronic inflammation, insulin resistance, and oxidation—that magnify the deadly potential of LDLs. Let this study motivate you to ask yourself, "How low can my LDLs go?"

HDLs: Aim Even Higher

High-density lipoproteins, or HDLs, whiz around in your bloodstream like squadrons of laser-guided vacuum cleaners, grabbing LDLs and hauling them to the liver for disposal. HDLs actually fuse with LDLs and remove their cholesterol cargo. New evidence suggests that HDLs also act as antioxidants, blocking LDLs from causing plaque-promoting damage.

HDLs are so potent that every one-point increase in HDL levels reduces heart attack risk by 3 to 4 percent; a high HDL level offers such powerful protection that it can even reduce the menace posed by other heart risks, such as overweight or diabetes. Low HDLs, in contrast, are dangerous because they leave your heart unprotected against LDLs and another damaging type of blood fat, triglycerides.

The latest news: In 2004, the American Heart Association raised its recommended HDL levels for women to 50 mg/dl, up from 40 mg/dl—a 25 percent increase and a recognition of the importance of this cholesterol-cleaning crew. Note that before menopause, women typically have higher HDLs than men; many experts actually recommend a target of 60 mg/dl for women.

Triglycerides: Push Down the "Other" Blood Fat

Triglycerides aren't a form of cholesterol, but because they act in a similar way and have similar effects, they are often grouped with cholesterol in any discussion of heart risks.

Triglycerides are bits of fat in the bloodstream that collect excess calories from the food you eat and whisk them away to fat cells for long-term storage.

Triglycerides can also become the raw material for LDLs, making them another dangerous actor in the heart disease drama. Newer studies suggest that triglycerides alone can predict heart risk, since they encourage atherosclerosis, especially in women. Recent research even suggests that too many triglycerides can form a roadblock in your blood vessels so the appetite-curbing hormone leptin can't send the "stop eating" signal to your brain when you've had enough lasagna. Belly fat and insulin resistance (for more on insulin resistance, see page 39) up your chances of having high triglycerides. Triglycerides are measured the same way as cholesterol, in milligrams per deciliter.

Smoking, drinking, eating too many refined carbs, and being overweight can all elevate triglycerides. On the 30-Minutes-A-Day Plan, you'll probably see your levels fall.

WHAT'S YOUR RISK?

LEVEL (mg/dl)	RISK
Under 100	Low
101–150	Normal
150–199	Borderline high
200–499	High
500 and above	Extremely risky

If you want high HDLs, though, don't follow Ancel Keys's prudent diet. A low-fat, high-carb eating plan will erode levels of these important fats, as will lack of exercise, smoking, and genetics. Look to good fats from foods such as olive and canola oils, nuts, and wild Atlantic salmon, along with regular, heart-pumping exercise.

#2 CHOLESTEROL: WHAT YOU NEED TO KNOW

Cholesterol is a waxy substance, produced from the fats you eat, that your body uses as the building block for cell walls, hormones, and a digestive fluid called bile acid. There are two types: "bad" LDLs, which form the basis of artery-clogging plaque, and "good" HDLs, which carry LDLs to the liver for elimination.

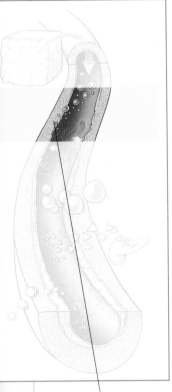

Excess LDL cholesterol burrows into arterial walls, forming the foundation for heart-threatening plaques that can narrow the artery and eventually break off.

HOW IT ACCUMULATES: Visceral fat, a diet high in saturated fat, and lack of activity can all prompt your liver to churn out more and more LDLs. A diet low in monounsaturated fat and a life devoid of exercise can deplete helpful HDLs, as can smoking and diabetes.

WHAT'S NEW:

New targets. Recent studies show that healthy LDL levels should be even lower than previously suspected, and healthy HDLs should be higher—especially for women, who have naturally high HDL levels prior to menopause.

Forget the "rusted pipe" theory of clogged arteries. Deadly plaque doesn't grow *on* artery walls, it develops in the walls themselves. LDLs start the process by burrowing through the inner lining of blood vessel walls. One type, small dense LDLs, is especially dangerous because it enters the walls easily.

Don't overlook triglycerides. This blood fat is checked every time your doctor performs a cholesterol test, but most of us overlook it. Don't. High triglycerides are linked to higher risk of heart attack, especially in women.

DETECTING IT: There are no physical clues to the levels of cholesterol in your bloodstream; only blood tests reveal their prevalence. A standard test, performed by your doctor, measures total cholesterol, LDLs, and HDLs, in milligrams per deciliter of blood.

STANDARD MEDICAL CARE: Americans spend $15 billion per year on cholesterol-lowering statin drugs, a number expected to grow by 25 to 30 percent per year as researchers recommend these versatile and effective meds to a wider audience. (At press time, atorvastatin, sold as Lipitor and made by Pfizer, was the top-selling drug in the world.) The next frontier? Better HDL-raising drugs. Many doctors now prescribe prescription-formula niacin to bolster HDLs.

VIABILITY OF SELF-TREATMENT: Very high for most people. One University of Toronto study found that a diet combining a range of cholesterol-friendly foods cut cholesterol levels by a whopping 30 percent in a matter of months.

High Blood Pressure

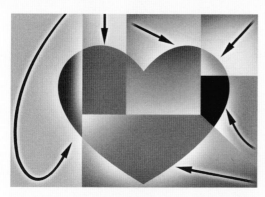

Imagine a peaceful river rolling placidly between cow pastures and cornfields. It rounds a bend and drops into a narrow, rock-walled canyon. Abruptly, the lazy current becomes an angry torrent, scouring the riverbank with sudden force.

Now imagine your own arteries—and

This is high blood pressure—a.k.a. hypertension, the grandfather of all cardiovascular risk factors, the original "silent killer" disease. Today, 50 million adult Americans (one in four of us) have it. If you're not in the club yet, just wait: Another 45 million of us have "prehypertension," the National Institutes of Health (NIH) warned in 2003. Odds are 90 percent that you'll develop this raging river in your blood vessels sooner or later. The odds hold true whether you're a man or a woman. While men under the age of 55 are more likely than women to have high blood pressure, once women reach 55, their blood pressure tends to catch up to and even surpass that of their male peers.

A gruesome 1733 experiment—in which the Rev. Stephen Hales, a British veterinarian and botanist, attached a thin brass tube to a horse's neck artery and reported that blood shot nine feet up the tube—first alerted Westerners to the fact that blood pressure was a force to be reckoned with. In the intervening years, an Italian physician developed a less messy, noninvasive way to check human blood pressure

their delicate, branching capillaries—growing narrow and stiff, a consequence of overweight, inactivity, stress, the doughnut and coffee you had for breakfast. Inside, unseen and unfelt, your blood hurtles along like a river squeezed into a stone canyon, banging so forcefully against artery walls that it can injure and weaken them. Ultimately, this pressure can rupture blood vessels in your brain (causing a hemorrhagic stroke) or your abdomen (causing an abdominal aortic aneurysm). It can also enlarge and weaken your heart and damage coronary arteries in ways that can lead to atherosclerosis—and perhaps even a heart attack.

(the oddly named sphygmo-manometer, a version of which is still used in doctors' offices today); insurance companies noticed that higher blood pressure was linked to earlier death; the first low-salt diet—a monotonous menu of plain rice and fruit—became the first blood pressure–lowering health food diet in the mid-1940s; and drug companies devised the first successful hypertension drug—a diuretic that, despite its beginnings in the era of the poodle skirt, is still considered the best first-line drug on the market today. In fact, a land-mark 2003 NIH study of 42,418 people with hyperten-sion found that these traditional "water pills" work *better* than newer, pricier blood pressure drugs—a finding that sent ripples through the phar-maceutical industry.

The Lowdown on High Blood Pressure

Despite all that knowledge, hypertension is still a myste-rious thing. Researchers are just beginning to understand how modern life and genetics team up to cause high blood pressure. Here are the most basic factors at work:

• **Your heart.** The harder it has to work (when you're shov-eling snow, for example), the greater the pressure on your arteries. When you're calm

High Blood Pressure

Blood pressure measures the force of blood against artery walls while the heart is contracting at full force and while it's resting between beats. For a super-accurate reading, see your doctor. Drugstore BP monitors are cheap and conve-nient but notoriously unreliable. If you use one, take three readings, then average them for best results. Here's what they mean.

BLOOD PRESSURE (mm/hg)	CLASSIFICATION
115/75	Ideal
Under 120/80	Healthy
120–139/80–89	Prehypertensive
140/90 and above	Hypertensive

(say, lounging on a tropical beach), your heart pumps slower, lessening the pressure on your blood vessels.

• **Your arteries.** Your arteries are lined with smooth muscles that can expand or contract as blood flows through them. The more "elastic" your arteries are, the less resistant they are to the flow of blood and the less force that's exerted on their walls. On the other hand, if you arteries are clogged by plaque, your blood pressure will naturally be elevated as blood is forced through a narrower channel.

• **Your kidneys.** They con-trol how much sodium your body contains and thus how much water stays in your blood (sodium retains water). More water means more fluid trying to cram its way through blood vessels—and higher blood pressure.

• **Your hormones.** So-called stress hormones cause your heart to pump faster and your arteries to narrow, which raises your blood pressure. Three other hormones—renin, angiotensin, and aldosterone—also team up to regulate blood pressure. The drugs known as ACE (angiotensin-converting enzyme) inhibitors lower blood pressure by controlling this trio of hormones.

Act Now

Luckily, experts are not only learning what causes high blood pressure but also what lowers it; you'll learn more about the pressure-lowering benefits of dark chocolate, great sex, and vacations later in this book.

While high blood pressure is a known killer—it plays a role in 75 percent of all heart attacks and strokes—one in three people with hypertension don't know they have it. Another one in three know they've got it but still don't have it under control. Out of sight, out of mind? Perhaps.

You may be ignoring your blood pressure, but the government isn't. The latest news? Lower is better, says the NIH. Forget the conventional wisdom that a reading of 140/90 or higher puts you in the hypertensive category. (The first number represents systolic pressure, the force of blood against artery walls during a heartbeat; the second number, diastolic pressure, is the pressure when the heart is relaxed between beats.) Now, a systolic reading of 120 to 139 or a diastolic reading of 80 to 89 is considered prehypertensive. The message: It's time to get serious about high blood pressure. To be considered healthy, blood pressure should be below 120/80.

Damage to arteries actually begins at blood pressure levels that docs have previously considered optimal, even stellar. Evidence gathered from 61 studies reveals that for most adults, the risk of death from heart disease and stroke begins to rise when blood pressure is as low as 115/75. After that, death risk doubles with each 20-point rise in systolic pressure and each 10-point rise in diastolic pressure.

Don't Discount "Accidental" High Blood Pressure

You gulped a travel mug of coffee in the car, sprinted across the parking lot—no time for a restroom break—and still barely made it to your doctor's appointment on time. Now you're in the exam room, and the nurse has just told you your blood pressure's a little high. Should you not worry, given the past hour's intensity?

Answer: You should still be concerned. You—and your doctor—should take this "circumstantial" hypertension seriously. New research from Indiana University School of Medicine, published in the *Annals of Family Medicine*, suggests that even one high blood pressure reading, regardless of the circumstances, is a preview of future heart disease risk and shouldn't be discounted by doctors or patients. Researchers checked the medical records of 5,825 patients treated for high blood pressure, then looked to see who developed health problems over the next five years. Those with a 10-point increase in systolic pressure during one office visit had a 9 percent higher risk of heart disease, a 7 percent higher risk of stroke, and a 6 percent higher risk of experiencing a first stroke or heart attack.

Perhaps the clearest, least mysterious thing about blood pressure is this: Plenty of do-it-yourself steps can help and are worth trying before you sign up for a diuretic or one of the newer BP-lowering drugs. Healthy lifestyle changes are worthwhile even if you're taking medication. From the eccentric (drinking tomato juice spiced with hot pepper) and the delicious (a cup of homemade cocoa) to the expected (losing weight significantly cuts blood pressure, as does limiting salt) and the mindful (relaxation helps, as does attending religious service), there are many small daily changes that can lower blood pressure. Losing just 10 percent of your body weight could normalize high blood pressure, without drugs. So could a diet rich in low-fat dairy foods, fruits, and veggies. And don't overdo acetaminophen or nonsteroidal anti-inflammatory drugs (NSAIDs), such as ibuprofen. Research from the Harvard School of Public Health shows that regular, frequent consumption of these painkillers raised hypertension risk.

#3 HIGH BLOOD PRESSURE: WHAT YOU NEED TO KNOW

Hypertension happens when capillaries—the tiniest blood vessels in the body, which deliver oxygen and nutrients directly to cells—become stiff and inflexible, prompting blood to rush through at greater pressure. High blood pressure in turn damages artery walls, making them more vulnerable to plaque buildup. It also weakens and enlarges the heart.

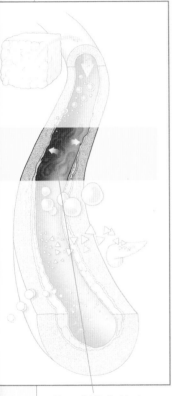

Excess fluid in the blood stream, coupled with narrowed or hardened arteries, can cause blood to flow with greater force, damaging arterial walls.

HOW IT HAPPENS: Genetics may account for 30 percent of cases of hypertension. For the rest of us, it's a combination of higher-than-normal fluid content in the bloodstream, due most often to an overly salty diet plus narrower, stiffer arteries—the result of atherosclerosis, inactivity, overweight, chronic stress, and/or diabetes.

WHAT'S NEW:

New guidelines. In 2004, the National Heart, Lung, and Blood Institute lowered its targets. The old advice that any blood pressure reading below 140/90 was healthy no longer holds; now, staying below 120/80 is the goal.

Damage and death risk rise sooner than expected. Evidence from 61 blood pressure studies shows that risks of fatal heart disease and stroke begin when BP is as low as 115/75. Risk doubles with each 20-point rise in the first number in a reading (systolic pressure) and each 10-point rise in the second number, diastolic pressure.

DETECTING IT: The only reliable way to measure blood pressure remains having a doctor or nurse strap that black cuff to your arm, apply a stethoscope, puff up the cuff until it cuts off blood flow, and measure the results as pressure is released. (Home blood pressure devices are great for regular monitoring, but you should also receive regular checks at the doc's office, where the machinery is properly calibrated and the results tracked over time.) High blood pressure usually has no symptoms that you can feel or see.

STANDARD MEDICAL CARE: About 24 million Americans take drugs to lower high blood pressure. The most popular are "water pills," or diuretics, which reduce the amount of fluid in the bloodstream. There are several classes of artery-relaxing drugs that are also widely prescribed, including alpha and beta blockers, ACE inhibitors, angiotensin II receptor blockers, and calcium channel blockers. Together, Americans spend roughly $15.5 billion a year on these drugs.

VIABILITY OF SELF-TREATMENT: Very high for most people. Dietary changes alone can act as a natural diuretic, lowering blood pressure as effectively as some medications. Meditation, exercise, losing weight, and quitting cigarettes also help.

Chronic Inflammation

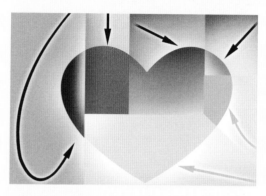

Slice your thumb while cutting a bagel. Slam the car door on your hand. Scald the roof of your mouth with the first bite of hot pizza. Your body's response? Warmth, redness, and tenderness—in other words, inflammation.

It's not a sign of weakness. Inflammation is a smart, take-no-prisoners defense mounted by your immune system to fix bodily damage fast and toss out intruders—germs, dirt, or toxins—before they can threaten life or limb. Any "attack" on your body—from cuts and bruises to bacterial or viral infections—triggers this rescue team, assembled by nature millions of years before the advent of soap, hot water, antibiotics, sutures, or hospital emergency rooms.

Your body's defense force is hard at work when you see or feel inflammation's trademark: a hot, red, tender spot. What you can't see: on the inside, an army of infection fighters called macrophages, T cells, and natural killer cells engulfing and destroying germs and materials that shouldn't be there, while squadrons of molecular "traffic cops" direct the immune system's well-choreographed work.

Inflammation has been a part of the human healing process since before the first people stood up on two feet, but this brilliant system may be doing its job too well for 21st-century humans. How? The problem isn't the short bouts of inflammation that fight infection or heal a shaving nick in a day or two. The modern threat comes from inflammation that can't turn itself off. This chronic inflammation—a response to overweight, sitting disease, aging, less-than-meticulous hygiene, low-grade infection, and the stress of modern living—attacks the very cells it intends to rescue.

The result is that your cells are under constant barrage by immune system chemicals. Recent research suggests that these chemicals help create plaque, the fatty gruel that grows inside artery walls. The chemicals also prompt plaque to rupture, spewing gunk into the bloodstream and causing the formation of blood clots that can stop a heart. At high levels, inflammation doubles or even quadruples heart risk.

Researchers have long known that inflammation plays a key role in conditions such as asthma, rheumatoid arthritis, multiple sclerosis, and inflammatory bowel diseases like Crohn's disease. Recently, though, studies led by Harvard Medical School cardiologist Paul M. Ridker, M.D., Ph.D., and others have linked it to heart disease and stroke, as well as type 2 diabetes and high blood pressure. Dr. Ridker and his colleagues have found that one marker of inflammation, an immune system traffic cop called C-reactive protein (CRP), is a better predictor of heart disease than cholesterol numbers. It may help identify the 10 to 20 percent of Americans who are at risk for heart attacks despite having healthy-looking cholesterol numbers.

The Inflammation Triggers

How can your body's "home security system" turn on you like that? Just as a sensitive smoke alarm is easily set off by smoke from frying onions or steam from your morning shower, inflammation is triggered by forces such as

Chronic Inflammation

C-reactive protein (CRP) is an immune system chemical manufactured by the liver in response to inflammation anywhere in the body. Measuring it with a $25 test can predict your risk of heart attack and stroke, detecting risk even in women and men with healthy cholesterol levels. To be tested, you'll need to see your doctor, since there are no home kits available. Ask for a high-sensitivity CRP (hs-CRP) test, which is the only one that checks for the levels of CRP associated with chronic inflammation. An older, "regular" CRP test, used for inflammation levels in diseases such as rheumatoid arthritis, isn't sensitive enough for this purpose. We recommend that you test twice. CRP levels fluctuate naturally and can rise significantly if you have a cold or the flu. Ideally, you should have two hs-CRP tests at least two weeks apart, then average the results. Here's what they mean.

You should also take your cholesterol numbers into consideration. Harvard Medical School cardiologist Paul Ridker, M.D., Ph.D., has found that looking at cholesterol and CRP together provides a clearer picture of heart risk. While your LDL levels predict how much plaque is clogging your arteries, your CRP number will tell you how likely that plaque is to burst.

LEVEL (mg/dl)	RISK
Under 1	Low
1–3	Average
Above 3	High

visceral fat, a glut of calories, the wrong foods, lack of exercise, and perhaps even daily stresses, such as a traffic-snarled commute. It's also turned on by low-grade infections, such as gum disease. Also, we're living longer than ever in human history; as a result, our bodies' aging tissues are exposed to inflammation's chemical irritants longer and

sustain damage more easily. Here are the details on chronic inflammation's biggest modern triggers.

• **Fast food.** A fat-packed, 910-calorie, fast-food breakfast of eggs and sausage on an English muffin plus fried potatoes flooded the bloodstreams of nine study volunteers with artery-damaging inflammatory markers, found researchers from the State University of New York at Buffalo. Levels were high for the next 3 hours. A fast-food diet could keep inflammation turned up indefinitely, researchers say.

• **Visceral fat.** Yes, that bad stuff again. Fat cells are now described by researchers as "hormone pumps." Among the chemicals they dump into your bloodstream are cytokines, inflammatory proteins that help direct the inflammation process.

• **Oxidized LDLs.** When "bad" LDL cholesterol particles meet free radicals in the bloodstream, a chemical reaction happens that makes LDLs better able to burrow into artery walls. There, they set off an inflammatory response that helps produce plaque, which is loaded with cholesterol, plus immune system cells and other substances. Inflammation then destabilizes the fibrous cap walling plaque off from the bloodstream. These "hot plaques" aren't always the biggest plaques in artery walls, but they *are* the ones most likely to burst and flood the bloodstream with substances that prompt fast blood clotting and ultimately lead to heart attacks or strokes.

• **Low-grade, chronic infections.** Influenza, bronchitis, herpes simplex, gum disease, a bacterium called *Chlamydia pneumoniae,* and another called *Helicobacter pylori* (the bug responsible for most stomach ulcers), all provoke inflammation and send inflammatory chemicals into the bloodstream. While we may not realize it, many of us live with these minor infections all the time; since they cause few symptoms, they go untreated. This discovery has lead heart researchers to investigate the use of low-dose antibiotics to cut heart disease risk.

• **Stress and anxiety.** Adrenaline, cortisol, and other stress hormones may turn on inflammation, too, say researchers at Ohio State University. Chronic stress may also impair your body's ability to shut down inflammation.

• **Choosing the couch instead of the walking trail.** Women and men who get regular physical activity have lower blood concentrations of CRP.

• **Not eating smart fats.** "Good" fats—found in nuts, canola oil, and some cold-water fish—are packed with omega-3 fatty acids, the building blocks for inflammation-*fighting* eicosanoids. Most Americans need more omega-3s and far fewer omega-6 fatty acids, which are found in safflower, sunflower, sesame, and corn oils. Omega-6s help your body produce inflammation-*promoting* eicosanoids. In prehistoric times, people consumed both types of fatty acids in nearly equal proportions; today, we get at least 11 to 30 times more omega-6s than omega-3s.

• **Too many trans fats.** These hydrogenated fats, baked into commercial crackers, cookies, breads, and cakes, interfere with the body's ability to produce and use "smart fats."

• **Skimping on fruits and veggies.** Skip 'em, as most Americans do, and you're depriving your body of antioxidants that help temper inflammation.

#4 CHRONIC INFLAMMATION: WHAT YOU NEED TO KNOW

Chronic inflammation occurs when the immune system's powerful defenses are switched on—and stay on. Doctors have discovered many things that can cause chronic inflammation in the arteries: everyday infections, such as gum disease or the stomach-ulcer bacteria *H. pylori*; substances released by excess tummy fat; and plain old aging.

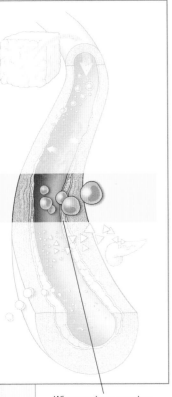

When your immune system is always in "attack" mode, one of its targets is cholesterol burrowed in arterial walls. One outcome is larger, more unstable plaque deposits.

HOW IT HAPPENS: Chronic inflammation is bad for the heart because it contributes to plaque buildup in the arteries. Here's how that works: When inflammatory chemicals discover LDL particles in artery walls, they send macrophages to eradicate the unwelcome cholesterol. The byproducts of this attack are foam cells that are the basis of plaque. As plaque grows, it develops a hard, fibrous cap, but inflammatory compounds can weaken this protective lid, making it susceptible to rupturing into the bloodstream. Other inflammatory compounds encourage blood to clot, and if constant, low-grade inflammation causes a steady supply of these compounds in your bloodstream, it can also lead to a heart attack.

WHAT'S NEW:

Predictive qualities. The link between internal inflammation and heart disease emerged only within the past five years or so. Now we know that chronic inflammation may help doctors predict which patients with near-normal cholesterol levels could go on to have heart attacks.

DETECTING IT: Doctors use a blood test for an inflammatory marker called C-reactive protein (CRP). Results under 1 mg/dl are ideal, 1–3 mg/dl is normal, and over 3 mg/dl indicates potentially chronic inflammation.

STANDARD MEDICAL CARE: So far, there are no drugs for chronic inflammation, although statins, beta-blockers, and low-dose aspirin may act as anti-inflammatories. Doctors are also exploring whether low doses of antibiotics are appropriate for people with low-grade, persistent infections.

VIABILITY OF SELF-TREATMENT: High for most people—but only if you take care of your whole body. Flossing, for example, is important to eradicate gum infections. Taking care of your digestion is important to minimize the bacteria that cause ulcers. Also, lose belly fat and eat more inflammation-cooling omega-3 fatty acids (found in cold-water fish such as salmon and in canola oil, nuts, flaxseed, and fish-oil supplements).

Metabolic Syndrome

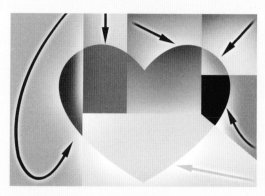

You can't see it. You can't feel it. But metabolic syndrome—out-of-whack body chemistry that may affect more than half of all American adults—quadruples heart attack risk and doubles stroke risk. The culprit: higher-than-normal insulin levels that you and your doctor may never, ever discover—until it's too late.

Unchecked, metabolic syndrome wreaks havoc with cholesterol levels, blood pressure, and blood clotting and can interfere with the normal, healthy functioning of artery walls in ways that encourage plaque to form. Metabolic syndrome also leads to type 2 diabetes and is now linked to infertility; cancers of the breast, prostate, and colon; and perhaps even Alzheimer's disease and kidney failure.

What's driving the rise in this little known and decidedly complex condition? A potbelly and a comfy chair parked in front of the TV. The numbers are rising in tandem with America's epidemics of obesity and inactivity. At least 47 million of us are believed to have metabolic syndrome, and some experts estimate that every overweight adult and child in America—64 percent of us— may have it.

The condition is a basic malfunction of the body systems that keep your cells supplied with blood sugar, their preferred fuel. Say you just ate a bowl of oatmeal. Normally, levels of the hormone insulin rise slightly after you eat a meal, persuading cells to absorb the blood sugar provided by your breakfast. In metabolic syndrome, though, the cells can't obey insulin's signal.

Why? Fat itself is the driving force. Researchers just recently figured out that belly fat—the visceral fat you've already read about—pumps some surprising chemicals into the bloodstream, including immune system messengers called cytokines. The constant flood of cytokines interferes with the absorption of blood sugar by muscle and liver cells. Basically, cytokines block signals from insulin to cells to let sugar in.

Now you've got cells that have no fuel and blood sugar building up in the blood-stream—two dangerous situations. Your pancreas responds by producing more insulin. Ultimately, the insulin overcomes the cytokines, and cells get the blood sugar they need.

For people with metabolic syndrome, insulin levels can rise two to three times higher than normal—and can stay elevated for decades. All that excess insulin is a setup for heart disease. It boosts levels of triglycerides in your blood-stream, lowers levels of "good" HDLs, and ensures that above-normal amounts of fat end up in your bloodstream after a meal and stay there longer. Insulin also morphs "bad" LDLs into smaller, denser par-ticles that can easily burrow into artery walls and form the bedrock for plaque. Addition-ally, it boosts concentrations of fibrinogen in the blood-stream, allowing blood to clot with greater ease. Small wonder, then, that metabolic syndrome is so dangerous for your heart.

But your doc probably won't be the first to mention it,

Metabolic Syndrome

If you have at least three of the following warning signs, you may already have metabolic syndrome; as a result, high insulin levels may be threatening your heart health more than you or your doctor realizes.

- A waistline that measures more than 40 inches for men or 35 inches for women
- Higher-than-normal blood pressure (130/80 or higher)
- Higher-than-normal triglycerides (150 mg/dl or higher)
- Below-normal HDL cholesterol (under 50 mg/dl for women or under 40 mg/dl for men)
- Fasting blood sugar test results in the: 100–125 mg/dl range. Doctors say people in this range have "impaired glucose tolerance," or "IGT" and are prime candidates for diabetes.

Other factors that raise your risk
- Overweight: a body mass index (BMI) higher than 25
- A sedentary lifestyle
- Being over age 40
- Non-Caucasian ethnicity (Latino/Hispanic American, African American, Native American, Asian American, Pacific Islander)
- A family or personal history of type 2 diabetes, high blood pressure, or cardiovascular disease
- Acanthosis nigricans: patches of thick, brownish, velvety skin at the neck, underarms, groin, or, for women, under the breasts
- Polycystic ovary syndrome, a female infertility problem
- For women, a history of diabetes during pregnancy

and you probably won't notice it on your own. There's no simple lab test for it, though suspicious doctors will use a three-hour glucose-tolerance test as an indicator. The only warning signs are a collection of *slightly* worrisome warning signs that, taken alone, may not even bother you or your doctor.

#5 **METABOLIC SYNDROME:** WHAT YOU NEED TO KNOW

This little known but widespread condition is linked to sustained high levels of insulin in your bloodstream. People with this condition have a raised risk for heart disease and heart attack as well as for stroke, type 2 diabetes, cancer, and infertility in women.

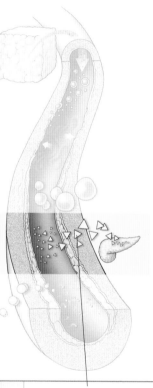

Abdominal fat releases a chemical that interferes with the absorption of blood sugar in your body. This causes a health-damaging buildup of insulin in the bloodstream.

HOW IT HAPPENS: This ultimate lifestyle disease is the direct result of too little exercise and too much belly fat. The two conspire to make muscle and liver cells stop responding to insulin, a hormone that persuades cells to absorb blood sugar. Your body answers by pumping out more insulin. The bottom line: Your cells absorb blood sugar, but insulin levels may remain dangerously high for decades.

WHAT'S NEW:

Metabolic syndrome can quadruple heart attack risk. It raises triglycerides, suppresses HDLs, keeps extra fat in circulation after a meal, and turns garden-variety LDLs into lethal small, dense LDLs that burrow more easily into artery walls. It also ups the risk of blood clots.

Up to 64 percent of Americans have it, but nearly all don't know it. There's no test and little awareness of this condition, which can lurk for decades before causing a health crisis.

DETECTING IT: There's no standard lab test that's widely available, although your doctor may detect abnormalities in the way your body handles blood sugar by giving you a glucose-tolerance test, in which you consume a sugary beverage, then have your blood sugar checked over a three-hour period.

Without a test, chances are good that you have metabolic syndrome if you have at least three of the warning signs listed on the previous page.

STANDARD MEDICAL CARE: Studies have found that some insulin-sensitizing diabetes drugs may help, but most of the 47 to 140 million Americans with metabolic syndrome don't even know they have it.

VIABILITY OF SELF-TREATMENT: Right now, self-care is the gold standard treatment for metabolic syndrome (although some docs have begun prescribing insulin-sensitizing drugs for it). Exercise—even a little bit—lowers insulin levels and boosts insulin sensitivity. Weight loss also makes your cells more sensitive to insulin, so your body doesn't have to pump out a super-size quantity anymore. Brand new research also shows that taking DHEA supplements may alleviate metabolic syndrome.

Oxidative Stress

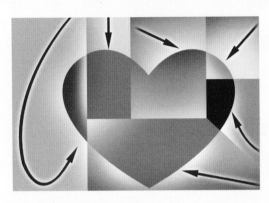

Two mysteries of the heart: Consider the lean, healthy marathon runner who, out of the blue, has a fatal heart attack. Consider also the overweight, fast-food-gobbling TV junkie whose cholesterol numbers are high yet who never, ever has heart problems. Cardiologists have long been

troubled by these two extremes of vulnerability and apparent invincibility.

What gives? One answer emerging from stacks of new research centers on oxidative stress—cell damage caused by roving molecular rogues called free radicals. Your body produces large amounts of destructive free radical oxygen

molecules through such round-the-clock processes as breathing and digestion. At any given moment, your bloodstream is filled with these molecules, whose destructive power stems from each having a single, unpaired electron.

The problem with free radicals is that they require another electron to balance

themselves out. So, like purse snatchers on motorbikes, these unstable particles steal electrons from other molecules in the body. This damages genes, proteins, and lipoproteins—and raises your risk for heart disease, cancer, and other diseases.

Normally, your body's own defenses—including antioxidants from the foods you eat—quickly mop 'em up. If, however, you smoke, are overweight, don't exercise enough, get stressed out, have metabolic syndrome, or order the large fries and cola instead of the side salad and grape juice, this cleanup doesn't happen. And it doesn't happen if your cells are pumping out extra free radicals while neutralizing the effects of ultraviolet light, pollution, toxins, too much alcohol, or even too many drugs, whether prescription, over the counter, or illegal. When your body's natural antioxidant defenses become overwhelmed, you've got oxidative stress.

Researchers now believe that oxidative stress is a key turning point for heart health, that it's the condition that switches atherosclerosis from "off" to "on." The decisive moment? When LDL particles are oxidized and can no longer deliver their innocent cargo of cholesterol to the cells lining artery walls. To your immune system, oxidized LDLs, which researchers call LDL-ox, look like grotesque invaders. Immune cells called macrophages trap them, and in the process, they become the fat-filled foam cells that form the foundation for plaque. LDL-ox also seems to make plaques grow larger and burst, leading to heart-stopping blood clots. High levels of LDL-ox can *double* your heart attack risk.

How powerful is oxidative stress? Some researchers, such as Ishwarlal Jialal, M.D., Ph.D., professor of pathology and internal medicine at the University of California, Davis, believe that without it, LDLs are relatively harmless. Following the misadventures of LDL-ox has also helped heart attack researchers identify circumstances that either protect LDLs from free radicals or leave them vulnerable. Here are the basics.

HDLs shield LDLs from oxidative damage. "Good-guy" cholesterol doesn't just ferry LDL cholesterol back to the liver for excretion. It also protects and repairs LDLs by safely siphoning off oxidized fats—yet another reason

to eat foods that increase HDL levels in your body.

If you have metabolic syndrome, your LDLs are more vulnerable to oxidation. As a result, you're more susceptible to heart disease. Even if your LDL levels are in the normal range, having metabolic syndrome raises the odds that more of your LDLs are the small, dense type easily damaged by free radicals. Sophisticated lab tests can tell you if you have these super-dangerous LDLs, but there's a simpler way to check. If you have low HDLs plus high triglycerides, you probably have small, dense LDLs as well. Even simpler: If you think you have metabolic syndrome, this is simply another reason to get more exercise, trim a few pounds, and eat fewer refined carbs.

Nurturing your natural antioxidant defense system is one of the most enjoyable aspects of the 30-Minutes-A-Day Plan. You'll get a rainbow of colorful, antioxidant-packed produce and juices at every meal, learn a timesaving secret that doubles the antioxidant value of veggies, discover a crunchy salad add-on that turbocharges your natural antioxidant system, and become a pro at picking the heart-healthiest treats at the farmers' market in summer and in the frozen-food aisle in winter.

You'll also learn the truth about the glut of antioxidant supplements on the market and why one of the longest recommended antioxidant capsules—vitamin E—won't help cut LDL-ox and could even compromise heart health. You'll discover soothing, 3-minute meditations and everyday yoga poses that let you build oxidation-busting calm worthy of a yoga master into the busiest of days.

#6 OXIDATIVE STRESS: WHAT YOU NEED TO KNOW

Oxidative stress is the term for damage caused by destructive oxygen molecules called free radicals. Our bodies produce free radicals naturally when we breathe, digest food, and neutralize alcoholic beverages and drugs of any type, and when cells convert fat and carbohydrates into energy. When free radicals damage LDL cholesterol, the stage is set for atherosclerosis and heart disease.

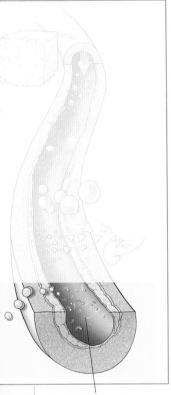

Excessive amounts of free radicals in your body damage genes, proteins, and other body cells by stealing electrons. This can lead to a host of heart-related problems.

HOW IT HAPPENS: Free radicals are usually eradicated by the body's natural antioxidant system. If that protective system is overwhelmed, free radicals begin to damage cells and other molecules, leading to atherosclerosis, cancer, mental decline, and other health problems. What overwhelms your natural free-radical stoppers: not enough fruits and veggies, too much stress, and too little exercise.

WHAT'S NEW:

Free radicals attack LDL cholesterol. This converts LDLs into a form that powers the development of atherosclerosis. The new form can also contribute to plaque bursting, and it's this burst plaque that can cause blood clots that block blood flow to the brain or heart.

The mind-body connection. Mental and emotional stress can boost oxidative stress; relaxation can lower it.

DETECTING IT: There is no test available to determine the level of oxidative stress going on in your circulatory system, but lifestyle choices pretty much tell the story. Overweight, a diet low in fruits and veggies, smoking, and lack of exercise all raise risk of oxidative stress.

STANDARD MEDICAL CARE: Americans spend nearly $2 billion per year on over-the-counter antioxidant supplements—vitamins E, C, and A and beta–carotene and selenium—intended to mop up free radicals. The trouble is, research has yet to prove they work.

VIABILITY OF SELF-TREATMENT: High for most people. Go for natural antioxidants: exercise, stress reduction, colorful fruits and veggies. Easy food switches that will turbocharge your daily antioxidant intake include sipping Concord grape juice instead of soda, sprinkling broccoli florets on your salad, and even eating canned veggies, which have twice the antioxidants of fresh. One supplement that shows promise is coenzyme Q_{10}, which may shield LDLs from oxidation.

Beyond the Big 6

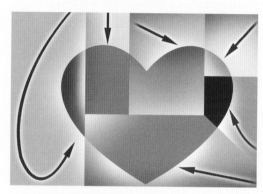

Molecular biologists and cardiology researchers are finding new heart threats all the time. These four are among the most proven, and powerful, new attackers.

1. Homocysteine

At higher-than-normal levels, this amino acid—created when the body breaks down proteins in the foods you eat, especially animal proteins—is related to a doubled risk of coronary heart disease. A Norwegian study of 587 women and men with heart disease found that mortality risk was eight times higher in people with high homocysteine levels compared with those with low levels of homocysteine.

The big, unanswered questions: Does hyperhomocysteinemia cause or contribute to heart disease, or is it simply a marker for some other condition? Does lowering it cut risk? Homocysteine may damage artery linings and promote blood clotting, but even the American Heart Association says there's not enough evidence yet to link it with heart disease—or to recommend trying to reduce it. Normally, your body uses folic acid and

vitamins B_6 and B_{12} to break down homocysteine for use as energy. While supplemental folic acid and B vitamins break down more homocysteine, it's too soon to recommend taking higher amounts than those in a good multivitamin and the foods you eat. Folic acid is now added to wheat flour in the United States and is found in citrus fruits, tomatoes, and veggies.

Are you at risk? Most insurance companies won't cover the $85 to $200 tab for a homocysteine screening test, and most of us don't need one anyway. However, if you have a personal or family history of heart disease yet lack any traditional risk factors, it may be worth a check.

2. Lp(a)

A renegade variation of LDL cholesterol, Lp(a) is an organic compound found in the bloodstream that can be a troublemaker for your heart. The particles have cholesterol cores and are robed in a sticky protein coating that seems to promote blood clotting. Lp(a) also binds LDLs more easily to artery walls, hastening the formation of plaque. High Lp(a) is an important risk factor for early atherosclerosis—over 10 years, it increases your heart risk by 70 percent, and it can exist in people with otherwise normal cholesterol levels. While there's not yet a treatment, knowing you have Lp(a) could spur you to compensate by taking heart-smart lifestyle steps.

Are you at risk? Lp(a) seems to be genetic, although in women, higher levels may be tied to higher body weight. If you have a family history of heart disease, ask your doctor about getting tested. While there's no standardized healthy level of Lp(a), one large study found that levels above 30 mg/dl doubled heart attack risk for women.

3. Nitric Oxide

This tiny molecule is a big player in heart health: It keeps blood vessels relaxed, which maintains healthy blood pressure, and discourages atherosclerosis by making artery walls more like Teflon so that white blood cells and clot-producing platelets can't stick. Nitric oxide, or NO, also suppresses overgrowth of muscle cells in artery walls, which keeps blood vessels from thickening, and it helps cut production of free radicals. NO is found throughout the animal and plant kingdom. It's the chemical trigger that makes lightning bugs flash their yellow-green lights on summer nights. Eating foods rich in arginine (NO's building block), such as beans, fish, nuts, and soy, can boost NO production, as can cutting back on saturated fat and getting up off the couch—all cornerstones of the plan in this book.

Are you at risk? Your artery linings produce their own supply of NO. If the lining's not healthy, production drops. (Another link: Low NO may be associated with higher levels of inflammation.) There's currently no widely available lab test for NO levels, but it's a good bet you aren't producing as much as you could if you are overweight, inactive, or a smoker, or if you have high levels of cholesterol, homocysteine, and/or Lp(a).

4. Apo(a) and Apo(b)

Think of apo(a)—a protein transporter that often ferries HDLs through the body—as the white hats and apo(b), which sometimes transports LDLs, as the black hats. You want more a's and fewer b's. One major study found that low a's and high b's upped the chances of a second heart attack. Researchers suspect these fat-plus-protein particles may be better predictors of heart risk than traditional cholesterol numbers.

Are you at risk? There's no widely used lab test for this emerging risk factor, either, but doctors are beginning to suspect that it may be a powerful predictor of heart health in women and in people with high triglycerides.

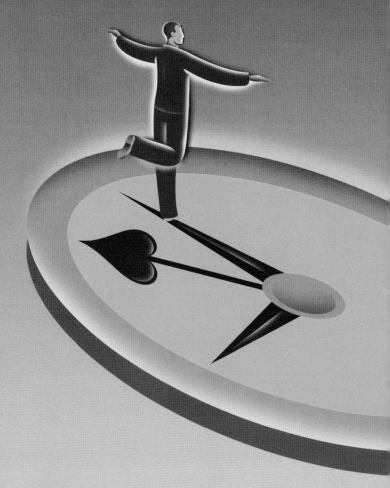

2 Welcome to the
30-Minutes-A-Day Plan

The path to a healthy heart is best traveled with small steps. Only this way does healthy living become simple, automatic, even pleasurable.

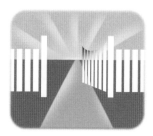

Our Promise

WELCOME TO THE 30-Minutes-A-Day Plan! First, let's start by telling you what the program is *not*.

- It's not one of those programs where you have to carve out 30 minutes of your day to do things that you would never otherwise do.

- It's not a rigid set of instructions to be followed to the letter.

- It's not a formal diet or exercise program.

- It doesn't have an expiration date. That is, it's not a 2-week or 12-week "intensive" that leaves you to face the world when it's over, as so many other health plans do.

Rather, the 30-Minutes-A-Day Plan can best be described as a promise: a promise that the time it takes to follow the heart-saving advice in this guide—advice that will wipe out *all* of the deadly heart attackers—will add up to no more than 30 minutes on any given day. In many cases, it may actually take less time or, even better, buy you some time to do other things you love.

Take the following before-and-after sample days, for example. You'll see that without drastically changing the structure of your schedule, you can sneak in lots of fat-burning, heart-strengthening physical activity, add eight servings of blood pressure–lowering fruits and vegetables, and scatter moments of stress-reducing fun and relaxation throughout the day.

And these examples barely scratch the surface of the heart-saving ideas and tools you'll find in the pages that follow. Integrate them into your life, and watch your cholesterol, blood pressure, triglycerides, and belt size drop as your heart health soars.

A typical Tuesday before the 30-Minutes-A-Day Plan

6:30 a.m. Roll out of bed, brew coffee

6:45 a.m. Shower, groom, get dressed, grab coffee

7:15 a.m. Wake kids, get them moving, shuffle them off to school

7:45 a.m. Go out the door

8:30 a.m. Park in nearest spot, grab coffee and pastry in café, take elevator to office

8:45 a.m. to noon Work, work, work

Noon: Grab sandwich with coworkers

12:45 p.m. Clean up, head back to office

1:00 p.m. to 3:00 p.m. Work, work, work

3:00 p.m. Grab a bag of M&M's

3:15 p.m. Fight afternoon slump

3:30 p.m. to 5-ish Wrap up day's to-do list

5:30 p.m. Drive home, listen to news

6:15 p.m. Nuke some mac 'n' cheese, go to kids' game/practice

6:30 p.m. Watch kids' game/practice

8:30 p.m. Supervise kids' bedtime routine

9:00 p.m. Collapse on sofa, nibble chips, drink soda, channel surf

11:00 p.m. Fall into bed

A typical Tuesday after the 30-Minutes-A-Day Plan

6:20 a.m. Roll out of bed, brew coffee

6:30 a.m. Shower, do 4-minute Healthy Heart stretching routine, groom, pour coffee with sprinkle of cinnamon, stash hearty carrot muffin and packed lunch in attaché to eat at the office

7:15 a.m. Wake kids, get them moving, shuffle them off to school

7:45 a.m. Go out the door

8:30 a.m. Park in farthest spot, take long way around building to far entrance, grab OJ, take stairs to office

8:45 a.m. to noon Work, work, work

Noon Round up coworkers for a walk

12:20 p.m. Grab prepared turkey and guacamole sandwich and fruit from office fridge, enjoy brief lunch with coworkers

12:45 p.m. Clean up, take stairs to office

1:00 p.m. to 3:00 p.m. Work, work, work

3:00 p.m. Stroll around office, catch some face time with coworkers

3:15 p.m. Have handful of almonds and raisins, wash down with water

3:30 p.m. to 5-ish Work, work, work

5:30 p.m. Drive home, pop in favorite CD, sing along

6:15 p.m. Open bag of prewashed spinach, toss into Tupperware container with canned salmon, baby carrots, grapes, drizzle of olive oil, splash of balsamic vinegar; add whole wheat roll, take off for kids' game/practice

6:30 p.m. Watch kids' activities while strolling around field or building, stretch on sidelines

8:30 p.m. During kids' bedtime routine, practice mindful meditation, absorbing sights and sounds as kids clean up and tuck in for the night

9:00 p.m. Sit down for favorite television show; do two exercises from Healthy Heart Strength Plan; during commercials, make next day's snacks and lunch

10:00 p.m. Wrap up next-day snacks and lunch, do 2-minute bedtime yoga routine, read book, or chat with spouse

10:45 p.m. Zzz

What You'll Find Ahead

We've organized our advice into six sections. Here's what to expect in each.

1. Eating Outside the Box

Here we present the 30-Minutes-A-Day Eating Plan—a guide to eating more of the foods that are most beneficial to the health of your heart. It's built around a simple, indisputable fact: Foods in their natural state are far, far more nutritious and healthy than foods that have been processed (hence "Eating Outside the Box"). We give you loads of advice as well as sample menus, cooking tips, shopping ideas, portion guidelines, and restaurant ordering suggestions to make heart-healthy eating as easy and delicious as possible.

2. Overcoming Sitting Disease

Sedentary living is downright dangerous, yet it's very easy to fix. We provide some of the simplest and most pleasant ways to get moving. Of course, there are walking suggestions—ways to sneak in steps throughout your day—plus easy, 5-minute strengthening routines and stretches and moves that feel great.

3. Nurturing a Happy Heart

You'll be surprised at the amount of scientific evidence there is that links happiness to heart healthiness. We can't order you to be happy, but we do the next best thing: provide clever, wise advice for adjusting your attitude and responses to stress in ways that help, not hurt, your heart.

4. Purging the Poisons

Not long ago, most doctors scoffed at the notion that common germs, chemicals, and everyday pollutants were harmful to the heart. Today, we know that living in a toxic world most certainly does affect heart health. Here, we give you the evidence as well as point you to the best ways to keep everyday toxins from affecting your heart.

5. Tracking Well

If you have a financial planner, you probably receive quarterly updates, and you know exactly which numbers to track to understand your financial health. It's a pity that doctors don't provide the same service.

In fact, most people don't even know what the most important measurements of health are. We'll tell you exactly what numbers you need to monitor to have a good picture of your health as well as what to track on a daily basis to make sure you're living in a heart-healthy manner.

6. Resources

From there, we provide even more assistance in the form of recipes, extra exercises, answers to common heart-health questions, daily tracking pages, resources, and more. Interspersed throughout are mentions of the many scientific studies that support our advice.

• • •

The 30-Minutes-A-Day Plan is a promise: If you follow the advice in our book, it will not only provide the most protection to your heart that you can possibly give it but will do so with a minimal sacrifice of time. Plus, the secondary benefits will be overwhelming: lower weight, greater energy, a better attitude, stronger immunity to everyday infections and diseases, and a far more positive outlook on life. So start the stopwatch and turn the page!

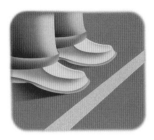

Getting Started

THE FACT THAT you've picked up this book shows you care enough about your heart to start making healthy changes for its benefit. As you'll see in the pages that follow, there are literally hundreds of tiny steps you can take every day that can add millions of beats to your heart's life. That's great news, but for folks who may not have given more than a fleeting thought to their health during recent years, it can also be a little overwhelming to tackle eating, exercise, and lifestyle habits in one fell swoop.

Here's a better plan: First, if you haven't already, see your doctor for a complete workup (see "Involving your Doctor" on page 58 and "Tracking Well" on page 205 for more on using your doctor as a partner), so you know what your heart status is right now.

Next, take the following quiz. See where you need the most help and start there. Once you feel confident in that area, continue with the other checkpoints until you've worked through all four.

What If I Need Help Everywhere?!

So you took the quiz and discovered that all of your lifestyle habits need a tune-up. Don't despair; that's why we wrote the book. If eating, exercise, and lifestyle all came up as high-priority areas, simply go through the book in the order it's written, mastering one section before moving on to the next. Or you can turn to the section that you feel is most easily tackled first, then work your way through in order of interest. Either way, the total time commitment is low, and the rewards are high. Get started today!

How's your diet?

1. **MY FAVORITE BREAKFAST IS:**
a. A bowl of oatmeal or raisin bran.
b. Two fast-food egg-and-sausage muffins to go.
c. Turkey on rye; I don't eat until noon.

2. **YESTERDAY I ATE THESE VEGETABLES:**
a. Broccoli stalks, baby carrots, red peppers, a mixed green salad, and some tomato sauce.
b. Corn and a salad with cucumbers and tomato.
c. The tomato and lettuce on my burger and a side of fries.

3. **WHEN EATING AT A RESTAURANT:**
a. I usually make some special requests, such as ordering sauces on the side or substituting baked dishes for fried ones.
b. I bypass the Alfredo and try to choose wisely, but I don't really know the difference between cacciatore and tetrazzini. I just go with what sounds best.
c. I'm there to indulge. Bring on the chef's special!

4. **FOR NUTRITIONAL INSURANCE:**
a. I take a multivitamin every day, along with a few special supplements such as calcium.
b. I pop a multivitamin most days, although I don't always remember.
c. I haven't taken a vitamin since Flintstones chewables.

5. **TO WATCH HOW MUCH I EAT:**
a. I dish out small portions at home and eat little more than half of what I'm served when eating out.
b. I avoid taking second helpings but still probably eat more than I should.
c. I have a hard time resisting seconds, and I usually polish off whatever I'm served.

IF YOU CIRCLED MOSTLY A'S
Your heart jumps for joy whenever you sit down to eat, knowing you always look out for its best interest by eating plenty of fresh produce, reasonable portions, and limited amounts of dangerous fat. Adjusting your eating habits is certainly not highest on your must-do list, but do page through "Eating Outside the Box" (page 65) for even more nutritional wisdom.

IF YOU CIRCLED MOSTLY B'S
Although your heart is often in the right place, the best dietary choices often elude you. Since you're generally motivated to eat well, with a little more know-how, you'll be a heart-smart diner in no time. Put "Eating Outside the Box" medium to high on your priority list.

IF YOU CIRCLED MOSTLY C'S
Put "Eating Outside the Box" high on your priority list; your current eating habits are harmful to your heart. By learning to make little changes, such as taking a multivitamin, trimming portion sizes, choosing healthier entrées, and even sprinkling cinnamon on your toast, you and your heart can live a longer, healthier life.

How active are you?

1. MY DAILY WALKING HABITS ARE:

a. I walk to the shower, to the car, and to the café at work. I'm too busy for much else.

b. I try to get up and move two or three times a day and usually take a nice walk at some point each day.

c. I usually try to walk for a few minutes on my lunch hour.

2. MY FAVORITE RECREATIONAL PASTIMES ARE:

a. Watching my favorite shows, reading, renting movies, and going out to restaurants.

b. Hiking, bicycling, and tennis; I like to be outside.

c. A good game of golf, but we usually take a cart.

3. IF SOMEONE SUGGESTED THAT I LIFT WEIGHTS, I'D:

a. Laugh; dumbbells are for muscle-heads.

b. Tell them I already do, two or three days a week.

c. Be intrigued. I know lifting weights is important; I just don't know how.

4. WHEN I REACH DOWN TO TOUCH MY TOES, I CAN:

a. Barely see my toes, let alone reach them.

b. At least reach my shoelaces; on a good day, I can graze the floor.

c. Reach my ankles, but I'm definitely not as limber as I used to be.

5. MY GENERAL ATTITUDE ABOUT EXERCISE IS:

a. Yuck; it reminds me of gym class.

b. It's the best part of my day.

c. I know I should do it, but it's the first thing I skip when my day gets busy.

IF YOU CIRCLED MOSTLY A'S

Dust off your walking shoes, sack your outdated images of exercise, and turn to "Overcoming Sitting Disease" (page 128). Inactivity is as bad for your heart as smoking, if not worse. The real news flash: Exercise doesn't have to involve drudgery or be time-consuming. Just a few minutes of easy activity a day can dramatically reduce your heart disease risk. Put it high on your priority list.

IF YOU CIRCLED MOSTLY B'S

Your get-up-and-go is great for your heart. By being active every day, whether by walking, volleying on the court, or hoisting dumbbells, you're keeping your arteries supple and clear.

Although you've already overcome sitting disease, check out that section when you've finished the others to learn more tips for fitting in the activities you love as well as adding new exercises to your repertoire.

IF YOU CIRCLED MOSTLY C'S

Try as you may, our sedentary society usually gets the best of you, sidelining your best-intended exercise plans. As you'll soon learn, a little bit of exercise goes a long way toward protecting your heart, especially if you can sneak in small increments throughout the day. Put "Overcoming Sitting Disease" medium to high on your priority list.

How happy are you?

1. **WHEN I TURN IN FOR THE NIGHT:**

a. I'm usually too wound up to fall asleep as early as I'd like. I'm a little groggy in the morning.

b. I sleep like a baby and usually wake up before the alarm goes off.

c. I'm a night owl. I usually hit snooze at least once, and I try to sleep in on weekends.

2. **I WOULD DESCRIBE MY TYPICAL WORKDAY AS:**

a. Somewhat stressful. There's a lot of pressure at work, and there's always too much to do in the evenings to really enjoy myself.

b. Busy but manageable. I usually carve out a little fun time for myself each day.

c. Awful. I dread Mondays.

3. **WHEN SOMEONE CUTS ME OFF IN TRAFFIC, I:**

a. Mutter a few choice words under my breath and seethe for a minute or two.

b. Shrug it off; there are always a few nutty drivers on the roads.

c. Get piping mad and sometimes shake my fist, or worse.

4. **I WOULD DESCRIBE MY SPIRITUAL OR RELIGIOUS LIFE AS:**

a. Fairly active. I may not make it to formal services as frequently as I'd like, but I take time to nurture my spiritual side.

b. Very active. I'm deeply involved in a spiritual community.

c. Nonexistent. I don't think much about that stuff.

5. **DURING A TYPICAL WEEK, MY ALCOHOL USE IS:**

a. A few drinks during the week, usually with dinner, but I sometimes overdo it on weekends.

b. Usually just a glass of wine with dinner, but sometimes I have two.

c. Not on a daily basis, but when I do drink, I like to cut loose.

IF YOU CIRCLED MOSTLY A'S

Life isn't bad, but it could be better. You fall into that frazzled no-man's-land of mortgages, car payments, job demands, and family responsibilities that can suck the fun right out of life if you're not careful. Turn to "Nurturing a Happy Heart" (page 164) early on and learn some quick, easy tricks for relieving your stress and replacing it with calm…or even joy.

IF YOU CIRCLED MOSTLY B'S

You have a smile in your heart most of the time. You've learned how to find calm in chaos and enjoy your life no matter how hectic it gets. By doing so, you'll lower your odds of developing heart disease in the long run. For even more tips on getting the most joy out of life, check out "Nurturing a Happy Heart."

IF YOU CIRCLED MOSTLY C'S

Like Atlas, you carry the weight of the world on your shoulders—and it's straining your heart. Symptoms of general unhappiness, such as high stress, anger, poor sleep, and alcohol misuse, elevate your risk of high blood pressure, obesity, and other heart-damaging conditions. Put "Nurturing a Happy Heart" high on your priority list.

How clean is your lifestyle?

1. **I USE TOBACCO PRODUCTS:**
   a. Daily; I'm a regular smoker.
   b. Not at all; I've never smoked.
   c. Not currently; I used to smoke, but I quit.

2. **MY DENTIST WOULD DESCRIBE MY ORAL HYGIENE AS:**
   a. Awful. It's been so long, he probably doesn't remember my name.
   b. Immaculate. Hey, I even floss!
   c. Pretty good. I'm a faithful brusher, but flossing and regular cleanings sometimes fall by the wayside.

3. **COME COLD AND FLU SEASON:**
   a. I'm sure to get hammered by at least one good bug.
   b. I get a flu shot and wash my hands like a surgeon.
   c. I try to avoid sick people, but I could do better.

4. **I WOULD DESCRIBE THE AREA WHERE I LIVE AS:**
   a. Congested, with heavy car and truck traffic.
   b. Rural; my nearest neighbors moo and give milk.
   c. Off the beaten path but not far from a large, more urban center.

5. **WHEN IT COMES TO GUARDING AGAINST ENVIRONMENTAL POLLU-TANTS SUCH AS LEAD AND MERCURY, I:**
   a. Don't worry about it; pollution is unavoidable.
   b. Keep up with reports on high-risk foods and drink filtered water.
   c. Keep a clean house and kitchen but don't take extra steps.

IF YOU CIRCLED MOSTLY A'S

It's time to clean house. You may feel that pollution, germs, and grime are inevitable, but with a few smart steps, the worst offenders are avoidable. Environmental assaults from tobacco smoke, viruses, air and water pollution elevate your risk of heart attack. Put "Purging the Poisons" (page 186) at the top of your priority list.

IF YOU CIRCLED MOSTLY B'S

If your heart were a linoleum floor, it would sparkle. By not smoking, protecting yourself during cold and flu season, and avoiding the worst environmental offenders, you keep your arteries running clean. For even more clean-living tips, check out "Purging the Poisons."

IF YOU CIRCLED MOSTLY C'S

Your approach to eliminating everyday toxins is a little like surface cleaning: All the countertops are clean, but don't open the closets! That's obviously better than not cleaning at all, but eventually, the covered-up clutter spills out and causes problems. Taking extra preventive steps such as exercising during low-ozone periods and getting a flu shot can not only protect you from environmental pollutants and germs but also greatly reduce your heart disease risk. Put "Purging the Poisons" medium to high on your priority list.

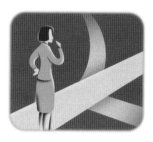

Staying With It

REACHING YOUR GOALS is exciting. After a few weeks on the 30-Minutes-A-Day Plan, you'll start seeing real results. You'll finish the day feeling as fresh as when you started. Your blood pressure will inch down. Those too-tight pants you'd banished to the back of the closet will fit again. Friends and family members may comment on your healthy glow.

Sooner or later, though, the new you will start being the status quo. When the hoopla of the new beginning fades, and the compliments become fewer and farther between, the real work begins. Studies show that half of the people who try to make healthy lifestyle changes start drifting back to their old ways within six months. Get past that point, however, and you'll have a habit for life. Here are 22 ways to stay motivated and make maintenance fun.

1. Wear your heart on your sleeve…or around your neck

We mean that literally. Consider wearing a heart-shaped pendant or finding some other visual trigger to remind you of why you're doing what you're doing. Here's why: "Motivation is not a constant; it waxes and wanes and is usually connected to an emotional response," says Howard Rankin, Ph.D., clinical psychologist for Take Off Pounds Sensibly (TOPS). "As you're sitting in the doctor's office, and he's telling you scary news about your blood pressure, you feel very motivated to change. As days pass, the motivation fades." To keep motivation high, you need a symbolic prompt to trigger that same emotional response. Wear a pendant or hang up a slogan like, "I want to see my granddaughter walk down the aisle," to keep motivating factors in focus.

2. Create a cheering section

When friends and family are behind you, you succeed. In an Ohio State University study of more than 900 men and women, researchers found that people are more likely to stick to their healthy lifestyle changes if their friends and families support and encourage them. Tell your spouse and kids that these changes are not always easy for you and that you'd love their encouragement. Even better, ask them to join you in some of your healthy new habits.

3. Create positive motivators

Fear of having a heart attack can certainly fuel the fires of motivation, but go easy on the doom and gloom, warns Dr. Rankin, because too much worrying can have the opposite effect. "It's human nature to avoid thinking about unpleasant things. If you constantly remind yourself that you're doing all these things so you don't die, you just might end up stressing yourself out so much that you quit," he says. A better strategy: Spin your negative inspirations to sound more positive—for example, "I'm packing healthy lunches and walking after work so I clear my arteries and build a strong heart."

4. Ask for help

Sometimes how you handle small roadblocks can make the difference between staying the course and veering off track. If you always make lunch for your spouse and he likes foods you can't resist, ask him to help you by making his own lunch. If piles of dirty dishes stop you en route to your evening walk, delegate the dishwashing to your kids. There's always a way around the little things, so don't let them get in your way.

5. Buddy up

Remember how, when you were a kid, you'd bang on every door on the block until you found someone to come out and play? When you finally did, you'd run around the neighborhood until the dinner bell rang. And if you didn't find anyone? You'd sulk back home and watch TV. We're not much different as adults. Company makes exercise and eating right more fun. It also gives you someone to be accountable to. If you're married, the best 30-Minutes-A-Day Plan buddy is probably your spouse. A Stanford University study found that men and women who took up exercise programs with their spouses were much more likely to be regularly active and much less likely to quit than those who tried to get moving without partners.

6. Track your progress

Using a chart to track your progress can be a motivational tool as well as a way to prioritize your heart-health goals. Each time you record your progress, you reinforce your commitment to healthy change. Listing daily activity or fresh produce consumed, as well as more general measurements of health such as weight, waist measurement, and blood pressure, can provide a very tangible reminder as your efforts pay off.

7. Find healthy friends

You don't have to ditch your carousing buddies or ignore old friends, but while you're trying to cement new heart-healthy habits, you'd be wise to limit contact with these people at times when you know they're most "dangerous," says Dr. Rankin.

For instance, hanging out in a smoky bar, drinking pitchers and watching the game, isn't going to help you quit smoking. "You may have to adjust your social circles by finding new, less tempting activities with your friends who maintain poor health habits, as well as spending more time with people who already embrace the lifestyle changes you're trying to make," he says.

8. Talk nice

Studies show that the more negative talk you use, the worse you'll perform at a given task. If you walk around telling yourself that you'll never change your ways, that you "just can't do it" or that you're "lazy," "weak," or somehow genetically disadvantaged, you're throwing in the towel before the game begins. Think of all the tough stuff you've done in your life: bearing and/or raising kids, working hard jobs, dealing with disappointments. If you could do all that, you can do this. Remind yourself of that daily.

9. Set instantly gratifying goals

Losing 40 pounds and lowering your blood pressure 20 points are good goals, but they won't happen overnight, and motivation can wear thin along the way. Keep those big goals, but set smaller, more quickly achievable ones as well. Small objectives throughout the day, such as, "I'm going to have a piece of fruit and two glasses of water before noon," are doable on even the toughest day and will keep you in a "can do" frame of mind.

Go easy on yourself. You are *making progress; you* are *a success.*

10. Think, "I'll just…"

When your motivation is so low you couldn't reach it with a 10-foot pole, lifting weights or preparing a healthy snack can seem like insurmountable tasks. During those low points, fall back on "I'll just" thinking. That is, "I'll just do my arm curls" or "I'll just get the berries out of the freezer." Once you take a step in the right direction, your momentum will pick up and pull your motivation along with it. Even if you don't do more than those little actions, you've at least done something to keep from going off the track.

11. Set up a reward system

Forward-thinking companies reward their employees with prizes as incentives for heart-healthy behaviors such as eating right and exercising. Do the same for yourself. Think of some goodies you'd like, starting small with something like a new purse or a boxed set of CDs or DVDs and working your way up to bigger and better rewards, such as golf clubs, kitchenware, or even a vacation. Then make your reward list, which could look something like this.

ACHIEVEMENT	REWARD
Exercise daily for one month	*Lord of the Rings* DVD boxed set
Lose 10 pounds	New shoes
LDL cholesterol 100 or lower	One week at the beach
Clean bill of health	New golf bag

Have fun with your rewards, and remember, they don't have to cost a thing.

You can take a Saturday afternoon to do nothing but lounge with a book or watch the game, or treat yourself to a day of window shopping in the city.

12. Give yourself credit

We have a tendency to dismiss the little things we do right, but all those little things, from choosing whole grain cereal in the morning to walking your dog after work, are at the heart of the plan. They add up to life-extending rewards—so give yourself a pat on the back every time you make a heart-healthy choice.

13. Have a fallback plan

Life is long. You're human. Inevitably, you'll hit a patch where you fall off the plan. If you prepare for the bad spells, they won't squash your motivation to get back on track. Decide now that when you see your waistline expanding or your blood pressure starting to rise, you'll get back on track by taking three 10-minute walks a day or eating a fruit with every meal. It'll help you get back to the program before you drift too far off-course.

14. Find role models

Everyone knows someone, whether a friend, family member, or coworker, who dropped eight dress sizes or stopped smoking and took up tennis after a bad brush with heart disease. Hold them up as role models: If they can do it, so can you. If you need more inspiration, talk to them; most people are more than happy to share their stories and suggestions.

15. Stop, think, act

Before you light that Marlboro or take that second slice of pecan pie, stop and force yourself to think about why you're doing something you know is bad for your heart. If the answer is "Because it feels good!" (and it probably will be), consider what else you can do, drink, or eat that may make you feel almost as good, then change course and do that. Before you know it, thinking before you act will become second nature—and so will making healthier choices.

16. Add variety

There are literally hundreds of tips in this book. When you find yourself falling into a rut (nothing kills motivation like boredom), look for something you haven't tried, such as a nice recipe or a fun exercise, and add it to your repertoire. The stimulation of trying new things will help spark your enthusiasm.

17. Donate your efforts

If you can't stay motivated to exercise for your own good, do it for someone else. You name the cause—from heart disease and diabetes to Alzheimer's and arthritis—and there's a charity group that organizes runs, walks, or bike rides to raise money to support it. Web sites such as www.active.com can help you find such charity events in your area. They not only give you a reason to keep moving, they give you the satisfaction of working hard to help others.

18. List the pros and cons

Anytime you're seriously considering quitting and going back to your old ways, take 2 minutes, draw a line down the middle of a sheet of paper, and list the pros and cons of your decision. This will help remind you of why you started in the first place and the consequences of turning back.

19. Find emotional outlets

Let's be honest: If what we eat and how we behave were nothing more than practical matters of fueling our bodies and taking care of ourselves, far fewer people would have weight problems or heart disease. We plow through a bag of chips or drink one too many glasses of wine not because we need the potatoes or grape products but because something is bugging us. We're bored, frustrated, anxious, or angry. Since those emotions aren't going to go away, you need to find other outlets, such as exercise, journaling, or relaxing hobbies, for those feelings, or you need to confront them directly rather than masking the hurt with unhealthy habits. "This is the real essence of maintaining change," says Dr. Rankin.

20. Take a vacation

Even if you love your job, you still need a vacation from its rigors now and then, right? The same is true of healthy lifestyle changes. Every now and then, take a long weekend, sleep in, and eat cheesecake. If you're true to the 30-Minutes-A-Day Plan the majority of the time, brief respites won't hurt your results and will renew your enthusiasm for making healthy choices.

21. Become an expert

If you're showing real progress, chances are you have found one or more aspects of healthy living that you really enjoy. It could be cooking with fresh foods or taking daily walks or doing yoga. Take that interest and explore it more deeply: attend classes, do it more often or for longer periods, or make it a hobby. There's no reason you can't become an outstanding chef, a master of meditation, or even a marathoner, once you set your mind to it.

22. Put your calendar to work

Too many of us do a poor job at long-term planning, particularly when it comes to the fun things in life. So change that. Make plans for fun, active events months away. Schedule an extended-family trip to the zoo for two months from now, a weekend away in the mountains for four months from now, a family outing to a major league baseball game in June, and a week of tropical vacation come next winter. Then make the reservations, buy the tickets, and mark the dates. This type of long-term planning not only gives you positive things to look forward to, but gives you motivation to get leaner, stronger, and healthier for the activities laying ahead in your life.

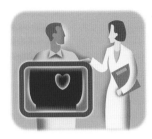

Involving Your Doctor

YOUR PHYSICIAN is a key player in your health life. He has the unique expertise to perform critical assessments, diagnose problems, and provide medicine and advice as needed to keep you well.

Your doctor is also very, very busy.

Surveys show that the average family doc sees three to five patients an hour, spending about 10 minutes—slightly more time than it takes to bake a frozen pizza—with each one. That's not to say that your doctor isn't good or doing his best job. It's just that no matter how competent your doctor is, there are hundreds of other patients lined up behind you, vying for the next 10-minute chunk of his time.

This is why you can't expect your physician to be completely accountable for your care. That's not his job. His job is similar to that of any other credentialed expert, be it a car mechanic, accountant, or attorney—to occasionally assess your condition, provide remedies when the situation calls for them, and detect trouble before it becomes serious. The rest of the time—which is pretty much all the time—it's *your* job to take responsibility for your health. That's where this book comes in.

You're In Charge

In these pages, you'll find take-charge advice that puts you firmly in control of your heart's health. What's more, you'll find advice that no doctor has time to give you, even if he were to spend twice or even three times the usual allotted time with you. Advice on calming stress, finding joy, and avoiding toxins—strategies that can slash your risk of heart attack. Advice on which fruits and vegetables are best for cleaning your arteries. How using some spices can lower blood fats. How stepping outside and walking down the block once or twice a day can literally add years to your life.

Doctors are trained in medicine; they know how to make you well when you're injured or sick by using drugs, splints, or surgery. Most are excellent at what they do, and many have begun to embrace more natural, lifestyle-oriented remedies such as good nutrition and exercise. But the truth is, not many are well versed in the lifestyle methods discussed in this book. There's an old expression: When your only tool is a hammer, all problems begin to look like nails. For doctors, the hammer is pharmaceuticals, which is why there were four billion prescriptions filled in the United States in 2004 and another five billion over-the-counter drugs purchased.

Again, we tell you this not out of disrespect for doctors. Rather, we want to emphasize the point that they shouldn't be the sole voice in your care. A doctor should be your primary advisor, but you should make the final decisions about your health.

This book will train you in staying well—and in getting better. Every tip we provide is grounded in scientific research. In fact, in a brand-new, groundbreaking study of nearly 30,000 people, German researchers discovered that taking simple lifestyle steps, such as those outlined in the pages that follow, could eliminate 90 percent of all heart attacks!

Go Team!

The best way to use this plan is in conjunction with your doctor's care. Following the advice in this book will probably make pills

It's Your Doctor, Not Your Mom

A healthy doctor-patient relationship is key to getting the most out of medical care. It's easy to blame rushed, brusque doctors if the relationship goes south, but in fact, we are just as often in the wrong. Our biggest flaw: not telling the truth. According to a report in the *Harvard Health Letter*, physicians routinely find that adults act like children once they get into the examining room by lying about behaviors such as smoking and drinking because they "don't want to get in trouble." Not good. Now that

you're an adult, the only punishment you'll get for hiding the truth is from your heart.

Tell your doctor *everything*. That includes embarrassing stuff that you should know better than to do, such as drinking too much, smoking, or even abusing prescription or over-the-counter medications. Tell him about all the pills you pop daily, including vitamins, minerals, herbs, and other supplements. Be honest about your diet and exercise habits. If you have some troubling symptoms or unusual health develop-

ments, share them, no matter how scary it may be to talk about them. Make a list and take it into the examining room with you.

Oh, and one more thing. If your doctor seems disinterested or discourages you from being an active participant in your own well-being, find another. There is no shortage of doctors who would jump for joy to see patients who are interested in taking charge of their own heart health. We know; we interviewed them for this book.

and medical checkups a smaller part of your life, but it is *not* intended to replace your regular medical care. You and your doctor are a team working in your heart's best interest. If you currently have high blood pressure, diabetes, or other heart disease risks, you absolutely must stay in contact with your doctor.

Whatever your current condition, even if you're perfectly healthy right now, we recommend that you set up an appointment with your doctor first thing for a baseline checkup. As you'll find out in "Tracking Well" (see page 205), there are a handful of medical assessments that speak volumes about your heart. You'll need to have your doctor get readings on these numbers, and he'll want to know them, too.

Indeed, the following is a list of routine tests that, based on current conventional wisdom, every healthy, health-conscious person should have. The timetable may be a little different for you, depending on your medical conditions. People in their sixties may find themselves going for tests each year, while those in their thirties or forties may get by with tests every two to three years. Discuss them with your doctor and set up a schedule that works for both of you.

1. Medical history/general physical

This is where you fill out a few double-sided forms, checking off every condition that you and your immediate family have ever had. Your doctor uses these forms to learn about your family history of heart disease and your general risk. During a physical, the doctor will also listen to your heart and check your pulse.

2. Blood glucose

Commonly known as "testing your sugar," this test helps monitor for diabetes (a major heart disease risk). After age 40, have your blood glucose tested about every two years.

3. Blood pressure

Since blood pressure is a strong indicator of the health of your circulatory system, you should have it checked every two years after age 40, or more often if necessary.

4. Cholesterol

This test measures the levels of good and dangerous lipids (fats) in your bloodstream. Generally, a checkup every two years after age 40 is sufficient, but if you're a man over age 45 or a woman over 55 or you have two or more risk factors for heart disease, you should have your cholesterol checked once a year.

5. EKG

In this painless test, you're wired to a machine that measures your heart's electrical activity. Some doctors recommend having one done once every year of adult life.

6. Stress EKG

This is an EKG performed while you exercise on a treadmill. Some doctors recommend having one every three years after age 35, but they're most important for people who have existing heart conditions. This test can uncover problems with heart rhythm or blood supply during exertion and can be used to determine how much exercise is safe for you, particularly during cardiac rehabilitation or after a heart attack.

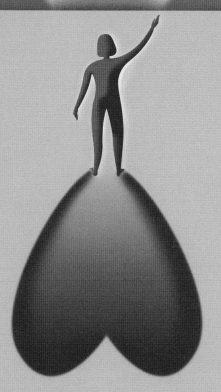

3 Eating Outside
the Box

*Few of us understand how powerful
the difference is between fresh food
and processed, packaged food.
One gives you health and
life; the other kills.*

The 30-Minutes-A-Day Eating Plan

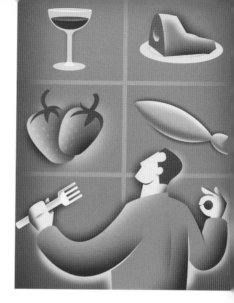

IF AN APPLE A DAY keeps the doctor away, what should you eat to keep the heart surgeon away—forever?

Try lean beef and a baked sweet potato, strawberries and a dollop of ice cream, dark chocolate, and red wine.

Thanks to cutting-edge nutrition research, heart experts now know that you don't have to give up your favorite foods in order to keep your arteries clear and your heart clean and well fueled.

In the pages immediately ahead, we're going to lay out the essential details of the 30-Minutes-A-Day Eating Plan. We suspect you'll be relieved by what you see: surprisingly few restrictions; plenty of inexpensive, widely available foods; and appropriate doses of moderation we're sure you can live with. We'll also provide lots of great tips for integrating the right foods into your diet and, in "Healthy Heart Recipes" on page 222, a whole host of delicious recipes featuring the most heart-healthy foods there are.

Don't stop reading when you get to the end of this chapter, though. In the pages that follow, you'll discover that the processed-food, restaurant, and weight-loss industries are working awfully hard to feed you unhealthy foods, and you'll need more than just the basics in this chapter to battle back! But as they say, let's start at the beginning: with the pillars of the 30-Minutes-A-Day Eating Plan.

- The five essential food groups for heart-healthy eating outside the box

- Sample meals that show you how to get all the essential foods without fuss

- How to adapt your diet if you want to lose weight

The Healthy Heart Food Groups

Here are the five types of foods that are essential to good health and the keys to a strong, long-lived heart. Base your diet on these, getting the number of daily servings we recommend, and your chances of heart disease will fall significantly—and almost immediately!

1 PROTEIN
Power for a Healthy Heart

No food group offers more versatile protection from the heart attackers than protein. Lean beef, eggs, and pork are packed with homocysteine-lowering B vitamins. Fish delivers omega-3 fatty acids that keep heart rhythm steady and discourage blood clotting. Skinless chicken and turkey are low in artery-clogging saturated fat, and their protein keeps food cravings (and the risk of overeating) at bay. Beans—legumes such as chickpeas, black beans, and kidney beans—are not only rich in high-quality proteins but are also one of nature's richest sources of soluble fiber, which whisks cholesterol out of your body and helps hold blood sugar levels steady.

Of course, no food group holds more peril for your heart, either. Cuts of beef and pork that are high in artery-clogging saturated fat raise your level of LDLs and your heart attack risk. The solution? On the 30-Minutes-A-Day Eating Plan, you'll find new meat cuts and proteins that will help keep your total saturated fat intake to about 7 percent of total calories. (Most Americans get about 12 percent of their daily calories

THE PLAN: PROTEIN

✓ **On the menu:** Fish, chicken, turkey, lean red meat, pork, eggs, beans (legumes).

✓ **Daily servings:** Three.

✓ **Serving sizes:** 3 to 4 ounces fish, poultry, and meats; 1 cup beans as a main dish, $\frac{1}{2}$ cup as a side dish; two eggs.

from saturated fats.) Here's how to enjoy heart-healthy meats and more.

♥ Create a seafood habit

The healthiest seafood for your heart is cold-water ocean fish because it's so rich in omega-3s. The most popular kinds are salmon and tuna; other choices include mackerel, herring, and anchovies.

Your goal is to get three or four servings of these fish a week. How? Have canned tuna for lunch twice a week (make your tuna salad with low-fat mayo) and salmon for dinner once or twice a week, or get anchovies on your Friday-night pizza. Or get creative: Use canned salmon to make salmon patties (we've got a recipe for you—see page 236), or make a Spanish-style salad of cooked potato cubes, sautéed onions, a can or two of tuna, olive oil, and salt and pepper. It's delicious!

While other seafood may not have as many omega-3s, pretty much all types are terrific sources of protein. So if sautéed sole or shrimp appeals to you more than salmon—or a chicken breast or steak, for that matter—by all means, choose the seafood.

Notice that the suggestions above don't require you to invest a fortune at the seafood counter or to do any type of exotic or challenging cooking. Today, there's not a household in America—no matter how far from an ocean—that can't easily add heart-healthy seafood to its diet!

That said, if you truly detest fish or have a shellfish allergy, simply substitute another type of lean protein—and consider getting omega-3s from walnuts, ground flaxseed, or fish-oil capsules if you can.

♥ Rediscover beef and pork

Long vilified by health activists, these classic centerpieces of the American dinner plate deserve a second chance—and a place in your heart-healthy eating plan. The fact is, both meats have gotten healthy makeovers to fit modern tastes: Beef is 27 percent leaner today than 20 years ago, and pork has 31 percent less fat. In one National Institutes of Health study, volunteers who ate lean red meat five to seven days a week had the same slight improvements in cholesterol—their LDLs dropped 2 percent, and HDLS rose 3 to 4 percent—as those who stuck with chicken and fish.

The lowest-fat cuts? Pork tenderloin, top and eye rounds marked "extra lean," boneless shoulder pot roast, and boneless pork sirloin chops.

♥ Shift the focus to beans

Beans deserve the lunchtime or dinner spotlight several days a week. Few people bother to learn bean-dish recipes, but if you can commit to coming up with three or four that your family enjoys, and then prepare one every few days, you will do wonders for your

Food Myths That Hurt Your Heart

Myth: *Shrimp is high in cholesterol.*
The whole story: It's true about the cholesterol, but it doesn't seem to adversely affect blood cholesterol, researchers say. More important: This popular crustacean provides healthy omega-3 fatty acids and is low in saturated fat. So dig in—boiled shrimp is a great choice at a party buffet.

Myth: *Eggs are heart attacks in a shell.*
The whole story: With 200 grams of cholesterol and 2 grams of saturated fat, eggs developed a reputation in the 1990s as forbidden foods for anyone concerned about heart health. Research shows, though, that for many people, eating up to two eggs a day *doesn't* raise blood cholesterol levels. Even better: Buy eggs enriched with heart-smart omega-3s.

Myth: *Extra-lean ground beef is a lean meat.*
The whole story: Ground beef may contain up to 22.5 percent fat and still be labeled "lean." One homemade quarter-pound burger may contain 7 grams of artery-clogging saturated fat. Instead, use skinless ground chicken or turkey breast, try veggie burgers, or pick truly lean meat such as extra-lean top round beef and ask the butcher to grind it for you.

health! Make meatless chili; create quick, hearty soup by mixing drained and rinsed canned kidney beans and frozen veggies with a can of low-sodium minestrone soup or chicken broth; sprinkle chickpeas or black beans from the salad bar over your lunch salad; or order a bean burrito (hold the cheese) when you go out for Mexican food.

2 GOOD FATS
Better Than Low-Fat

Why keep spreading saturated-fat-laden butter or crunching on snacks packed with artery-damaging trans fatty acids when you could eat as if you spent your days beside the Mediterranean Sea—spreading fruity olive oil on crusty bread and fresh veggies and snacking on almonds? Countless studies have shown that these cornerstones of the Mediterranean diet protect your heart. That's why nuts, olive oil, and heart-healthy canola oil, which contains some omega-3 fatty acids, get top billing in this plan, too.

All three are rich in monounsaturated fats. Eat them in place of saturated fats, and they'll lower LDLs, slightly increase HDLs, and reduce triglycerides. While you need to keep saturated fats low, monounsaturated fats can make up 20 percent of your daily calories. Just watch your portions—oils, nuts, and nut butters are calorie dense, so a little goes a long way. Here's how to rebalance your fat budget.

💜 Say no to saturated fats

Remove skin from chicken and turkey before eating; trim excess fat from all meats; choose mayonnaise and salad dressings with no more than 1 gram of saturated fat per tablespoon (look for versions made with canola oil, often at health food stores); and replace heavy cream in recipes with condensed skim milk. For baking and cooking, substitute canola or olive oil for butter by using one-fourth less oil than the amount of butter called for in a recipe (for example, in a muffin recipe, use ¾ tablespoon of oil instead of 1 tablespoon of butter). If you

✓ **On the menu:** Olive oil, canola oil, nuts.

✓ **Daily servings:** One to three of each.

✓ **Serving sizes:** ½ to 1 tablespoon oil; 1 ounce nuts.

must have butter, whipped varieties have 30 percent less saturated fat.

💜 Banish trans fats

Eat only packaged snacks and baked goods with no partially hydrogenated fats or oils listed as ingredients. Switch to trans fat–free margarine or use olive oil instead. (For more on why, see "It's All in the Processing" on page 78.)

💜 Pump up the monounsaturated fats

Invest in an olive-oil sprayer (Misto is one brand) to give toast and veggies a light, flavorful coating instead of using butter or margarine. Make olive and canola oils your first choices for salad dressings, marinades, and cooking. (Other oils have lower levels of heart-healthy monos.) Try olive oil for scrambling eggs, browning stew or soup meat, and sautéing vegetables. Commercial olive or canola oil sprays are good for coating cookware to prevent sticking.

💜 Goodbye, Mr. Chips—hello, nuts

The monounsaturated fats in nuts (and omega-3s in walnuts) make these delicious nuggets a perfect heart-healthy snack. To guard against overeating, put one serving in a bowl, put the container back in the cupboard, then enjoy. Choose unsalted nuts to help control blood pressure.

Diversify your nut portfolio

Beyond peanuts and walnuts, try pistachios, pecans, and hazelnuts. Sprinkle them on cereal and salads and add them to muffin batter, yogurt, and pudding.

Don't forget the peanut butter

PB has impressive amounts of monounsaturated fat, protein, vitamin E, and fiber. Have some on toast for breakfast, enjoy a good old PB&J for lunch (on whole wheat bread, of course), or scoop out a tablespoon and use it as a dip for baby carrots, apple slices, or pears as an afternoon snack.

Top desserts with Coromega

This orange-flavored, pudding-like gel (you can eat it straight from a single-serving container or spoon it over yogurt or ice cream) is about as far as you can get from fish in taste, but it's packed with the omega-3s usually found in seafood. Find more info about this emulsified form of omega-3 fatty acids, produced by the Coromega Company of Carlsbad, California, at www.coromega.com or by calling (877) 275-3725.

3 FRUIT AND VEGETABLES
Nature's Cholesterol Cure

Our ancestors filled their bellies with wild produce; today, researchers suspect that our bodies evolved to expect big daily doses of the antioxidants, cholesterol-lowering phytosterols, and soluble fiber found in fruits and vegetables. Without them—and most of us get four produce servings a day or less—heart risk rises. Here's how to hunt and gather nine servings a day at home and at work.

THE PLAN: FRUITS AND VEGETABLES

✓ **On the menu:** Any and all produce.

✓ **Daily servings:** Three or four of fruit; four or five of vegetables.

✓ **Serving sizes:** 1 medium fruit; $1/2$ cup raw, cooked, canned, or frozen fruit or vegetables; 6 ounces 100 percent fruit or vegetable juice; 1 cup raw leafy greens; $1/4$ cup dried fruit.

Take a juice break

Sip 100 percent orange juice or Concord grape juice as one of your daily fruit servings, or mix juice concentrate with olive oil for a sweet salad dressing.

Whirl up a blender drink

Toss frozen strawberries; orange juice; and a banana, pear, or nectarine (take the pit out first!) into the blender for a triple serving of fruit, smoothie-style. Add plain yogurt with a sprinkle of wheat germ or ground flaxseed, and you've got breakfast.

Chop early, grab often

Buy a cantaloupe or small watermelon, cube the fruit, and keep it in a container in the fridge for an easy, antioxidant-rich snack when you're looking for something to nosh on.

Put fruit and veggies in easy reach

Keep a bowl of cherry tomatoes and a bowl of bananas or apples on the kitchen counter. If you see them, you'll eat them.

Redefine fast food

Supermarkets have a huge selection of bagged salad greens. In 15 minutes, you can grab a bag (look for extras, such as cranberries and walnuts right in the bag) of baby spinach or chopped romaine and a container of tomatoes, sliced carrots, mandarin orange slices, chopped nuts, and a sprinkle of raisins from the salad bar. You'll have five produce servings right there!

🍇 Obey a new second-helpings rule

Allow yourself to take second helpings only of vegetables at dinner. You'll save calories from fat and boost fiber intake.

🍇 Eat the rainbow

From blueberries to carrots and tomatoes to pineapple, have as many different-colored fruits and veggies as possible each day to get the widest variety of nutrients.

🍇 Splurge like a chef

You'd buy a fancy cake, a specialty ice cream, or a cheese-covered frozen veggie, so why not those gorgeous raspberries, that box of clementines, or a bunch of deep green asparagus instead?

🍇 Buy insurance for your cupboard and freezer

This means canned (in juice) and frozen fruit and veggies for times when you run out of fresh or don't have time to wash and chop. Some frozen produce has more nutrients than the fresh stuff because it's frozen immediately after harvesting.

🍇 Tuck extras in

Keep a bag of grated carrots in the fridge to toss into soups, stews, casseroles, sauces, tuna salad, and even muffins. Add extra frozen veggies to soups and stews.

🍇 Wash and blot, but don't peel

Cut your risk of food poisoning by washing all produce and blotting it dry. Then eat it all, skin included—it's full of fiber, and the fruit or veggie flesh just below it contains extra nutrients.

4 WHOLE GRAINS
Count These Carbs In

Simply eating a high-fiber, whole grain breakfast could cut your risk of heart attack by 15 percent; switching completely from refined to whole grains could slash it by 30 percent. That's the power of whole grains. These natural nuggets are filled with vitamin E and a wealth of heart-protecting phytochemicals, plus insoluble fiber to help digestion. Some, such as barley and oatmeal, also have cholesterol-lowering soluble fiber.

In the following chapter, you'll learn more about grain processing and why refined grains aren't nearly as healthy for you as whole grains. For now, here's how to fit in three or more whole grains every day.

🍇 Think fiber in the morning

Here's new motivation to breakfast on oatmeal or another high-fiber cereal: Each gram of soluble fiber cuts your LDLs by as

---

THE PLAN: WHOLE GRAINS

✓ **On the menu:** Whole wheat bread, pasta, barley, bulgur, and couscous; brown rice; whole grain and high-fiber cereals, including oatmeal.

✓ **Daily servings:** Two to four.

✓ **Serving sizes:** 1 slice bread; $1/2$ cup rice, pasta, barley, bulgur, or couscous; $1/2$ to $1^1/2$ cups cereal (varies with brand).

much as 2 points, according to the American Heart Association. From raisin bran with 8 grams per serving to supercharged fiber cereals with as many as 14 grams, there are lots of cholesterol warriors in the cereal aisle. One bowl a day could lower your LDLs by 16 to 28 points.

💟 Boil once, then freeze the leftovers

Brown rice, barley, and bulgur are delicious. To save weekday prep time, cook up a big pot on the weekend and freeze extras in single-meal portions, then defrost in the microwave as needed. Add to ground poultry for extra body when making meat loaf or burgers.

💟 Use the rule of three

Choose breads with "whole wheat" leading the ingredients list and with 3 grams of fiber per serving. Substitute whole wheat toast for bagels and low-fat multigrain muffins for pastries. Make sandwiches with whole grain breads or rolls.

5 DAIRY FOODS
Better Blood Pressure Control

Having milk on your morning cereal, a cup of yogurt as a midafternoon snack, and grated low-fat cheese on your chili at dinnertime boosts your intake of calcium, a mineral vital for healthy blood pressure. In the landmark study, Dietary Approaches to Stop Hypertension (DASH), a healthy diet that included low-fat milk products cut blood pressure levels as effectively as drugs. Researchers suggest that dairy's calcium and protein work with the magnesium, potassium, and fiber in fruits, veggies, and whole

---

THE PLAN: DAIRY FOODS

✓ **On the menu:** Low-fat or fat-free milk, yogurt, cheese, even ice cream.

✓ **Daily servings:** Two to three.

✓ **Serving sizes:** 8 ounces milk; 1 ounce low-fat, low-sodium cheese; 1 cup yogurt; low-fat ice cream.

---

grains to better regulate blood pressure. Use the following tips to get the calcium advantage without adding saturated fat.

💟 Ease into fat-free

If you drink whole or 2% milk, switch to low-fat for a while, then try fat-free. Or use fat-free milk in cereal and soups, where the flavor difference is less noticeable, and use low-fat in coffee and hot cocoa.

💟 Add fruit

A cup of yogurt topped with chopped fruit and a tablespoon of nuts makes a filling snack. Try vanilla yogurt topped with banana slices and a dusting of cinnamon; add sliced strawberries and chopped walnuts to strawberry yogurt.

💟 Replace the water

Use milk instead when cooking oatmeal or soups that can be served creamed.

💟 Top it with cheese

An ounce of grated low-fat cheese is delicious melted on bread or as a topping for chili or beans.

Healthy Heart Sample Meals

Now that you know the foods that make up the 30-Minutes-A-Day Eating Plan, we'll show you how to get them on your plate. No long lecture here—just lots of sample meals, with the right portion sizes, for you to try.

BREAKFASTS

Here are eight breakfasts to choose from. Each is 300 to 500 calories.

1. Yogurt and Muffin Morning

- 1 cup mixed *fresh fruit* (melon, banana, apple, berries) topped with 1 cup light vanilla *yogurt* and ⅓ cup toasted *almonds*
- 1 small *bran muffin*
- 1 cup *fat-free milk*

2. Oatmeal and Fruit

- 1 cup old-fashioned *oatmeal* with 1 to 2 Tbsp ground flaxseed or wheat germ; ½ cup low-fat or fat-free milk; and ¼ cup raisins or ½ cup sliced strawberries, bananas, or juice-packed canned peaches (men: add 1 slice whole wheat toast with 1 Tbsp trans fat–free margarine)

3. Morning Cheese Melt

- 1 whole wheat *English muffin* topped with 1 oz (2 oz for men) low-fat, low-sodium cheese and toasted in a toaster oven until cheese melts
- 1 orange, peach, apple, or pear

4. Cereal-Plus Breakfast

- 1 cup *high-fiber cereal* (at least 7 grams fiber per serving) with ½ cup low-fat or *fat-free milk*, 2 Tbsp chopped *walnuts*, and 1 cup *blueberries*

5. PB&B Sandwich

- 1 slice *whole wheat bread* spread with 1 Tbsp *peanut butter* (2 Tbsp for men) and topped with *sliced banana*
- 1 cup low-fat or *fat-free milk*

6. Breakfast Trail Mix

- Combine 1 cup *whole grain cereal*, ¼ cup *nuts*, and ¼ cup *dried fruit*
- 1 cup low-fat or *fat-free milk*

7. Smoothie

- In a blender or food processor, mix together 1 cup *orange juice*, ½ cup frozen *strawberries*, and 1 cup low-fat *vanilla or plain yogurt*.
- 1 slice *whole wheat toast* with 1 Tbsp trans fat–free margarine (2 slices for men)

8. Vegetable Omelet

- Cook 2 *well-beaten eggs* in ½ tsp olive oil in a nonstick skillet. When firm, add ½ oz grated low-fat, low-sodium *cheese* plus sliced *mushrooms, tomato, green bell pepper, and onion*.
- 1 slice *whole grain toast* (2 for men) with 1 Tbsp trans fat–free margarine

LUNCHES

Here are seven lunches, each in the 500-calorie range. All are healthy and delicious.

1. Soup and Salad

- For the soup: Heat canned low-sodium *Italian minestrone* with ½ cup frozen green beans and ½ cup canned kidney beans (drained and rinsed).

- For the salad: Top *mixed baby greens* (rinse bagged greens) with ¼ avocado; ½ pear, sliced; ½ cup chopped red bell pepper; and chopped red onion to taste; toss with 1 tablespoon olive oil dressing.

- 1 small *whole wheat roll* or 1 slice whole grain bread

2. Havin' Some Salmon!

- Your choice of...
  Salmon salad on pita: Mix 4 oz canned salmon with 2 Tbsp each chopped walnuts, green onion, red bell pepper, and grated carrot; 1 Tbsp light mayo; and 1 tsp mustard, then spoon into a small whole wheat pita.

or...

Easy salmon melt: Mix 4 oz salmon with 2 Tbsp chopped celery and grated carrot and 1 Tbsp light mayo. Divide evenly between 2 whole wheat English muffin halves, top each with ½ oz low-fat cheddar or American cheese, and broil until cheese bubbles.

3. Wrapping Mexican Style

- *Bean burrito:* Mix ⅓ cup canned pinto beans (drained, rinsed, and smashed), with 4 Tbsp shredded low-fat cheddar cheese and 3 Tbsp salsa, then roll in a warmed 8" tortilla or spoon into a whole wheat pita.

- 1 cup *baby carrots*

- 1 piece whole *fruit* or 1 cup berries

4. Poultry Options

- Your choice of...
  Chicken salad wrap: Combine chopped precooked chicken breast strips with shredded coleslaw vegetables and low-fat honey mustard dressing. Spread

Workday Snacks

Resist the candy machine! Stash these sweet, savory, crunchy, and downright indulgent munchies in your desk drawer, briefcase, or office fridge. To double the heart protection, take one of these snacks along on an afternoon stroll around your office building.

Nuts. Fill small zipper-lock bags with 1-ounce portions—24 almonds, 14 walnut halves, 18 cashews, or 50 pistachios (in the shell).

Dried fruit. Bag up ¼-cup portions of raisins, dried apricots, dried cranberries, and even dried plums (the new name for prunes).

Single-serving fruit. Canned fruit in its own juice or light syrup is available in containers with pull-off lids. Don't forget to pack a plastic spoon!

Whole-grain, trans fat–free crackers. Store in a zipper-lock bag to keep them fresh. About four crackers make a healthy, good-size snack.

Fresh fruit, low-fat yogurt, single-serving cans of Concord grape juice, string cheese, or mozzarella sticks. Pack any of these into a lunch-size cooler bag, put your name on it, and stash it in the office refrigerator.

cranberry relish on a low-fat tortilla, spoon on the chicken salad, and roll up. or...

Turkey and avocado sandwich: Spread 2 slices whole grain bread with honey mustard and layer with sliced lean turkey breast; $1/4$ avocado, sliced (or 1 Tbsp guacamole); and 2 thick slices tomato.

5. Veggie Burger

- Pan-fry or grill a *veggie patty* and serve on a whole grain bun with 3 large leaves romaine lettuce, 2 thick slices tomato, and 2 Tbsp honey mustard.

- 12 *baby carrots*

6. Peanut Butter Sandwich Deluxe

- Spread 2 Tbsp *peanut butter* on 1 slice *whole grain bread*; top with *raisins* and sliced banana or a thin layer of *strawberry jam* and sliced strawberries.

- *Cherry tomatoes*

- *Baby carrots*

7. Leftover Makeover

- Arrange leftover *chicken, fish, beef, or beans* on a bed of rinsed *baby spinach or field greens* and top with sliced carrots, cherry tomatoes, and 1 to 2 Tbsp almonds; drizzle with olive oil dressing.

- 1 small *whole wheat roll* or 1 slice whole grain bread

DINNERS

Here are seven choices. Each is about 600 calories—more than enough to be satisfying and filling.

1. Salmon and Salad

- Your choice of...
  broiled or *grilled salmon* (4-ounce piece)
  or...
  Lemony Salmon Patties (recipe on page 236)

- *Quick spinach salad:* Rinse prewashed baby spinach and top with presliced car-

Heart-Smart Toppings

For both flavor and health, add the following liberally to cereal, sauces, soups, salads, stir-fries, and roasts.

Ground flaxseed. This is the richest plant source of heart-protecting omega-3 fatty acids. Buy preground or milled flax and store it in the freezer, or look for a flax mill loaded with flaxseeds at a kitchen store. Add 1 to 2 tablespoons to food.

Chopped nuts. Add 1 to 2 tablespoons to cereal, salads, or fruit for extra fiber and

monounsaturated fat (walnuts also provide omega-3s). Chopped nuts stay fresh longer in the freezer.

Wheat germ. It's a terrific natural source of vitamin E, an antioxidant that may discourage artery-clogging plaque. Add 1 to 2 tablespoons per serving to cereal and baked goods. Store in the fridge or freezer to preserve freshness.

Cinnamon. Just $1/2$ teaspoon a day can help control blood sugar and lower cholesterol.

Sprinkle some in coffee, cereal, and fruit salad.

Grated ginger. Add this powerful antioxidant to meat dishes, fruit, and desserts. You can keep some fresh ginger in the freezer and simply grate what you need, or use powdered ginger.

Chopped garlic. This beloved flavoring may lower cholesterol. Add it to salad dressings, meat dishes, veggies, and sauces. Store prechopped garlic in the fridge.

rots, cherry tomatoes, a handful of pre-chopped walnuts, and a handful of cranberries; toss with 1 Tbsp dressing made with ½ Tbsp olive oil, ½ Tbsp orange juice concentrate, and ½ tsp salt.

- ½ cup *brown rice*, whole wheat *couscous*, or *barley*, or 1 slice *whole grain bread*

2. New Twists on Poultry

- Your choice of ...
  Zesty Apricot Turkey (recipe on page 237)
  or...
  Herbed Lime Chicken (recipe on page 238)
  or...
  Cranberry Chicken (recipe on page 238)
- 1 baked *sweet potato*
- *Cauliflower Provençal* (recipe on page 232)
- Sliced *red bell pepper* rings

3. Here's the Beef

- Your choice of...
  grilled or broiled bottom, eye, or top round; round tip; top sirloin; top loin; or tenderloin (4-ounce piece)
  or...
  Beef kabobs: Mix olive oil, balsamic vinegar, and chopped garlic to marinate (or brush on) beef cubes, red bell pepper pieces, onion chunks, and cherry tomatoes; place veggies and beef on skewers and grill or broil until beef is done.

Two Perfect Pizzas

You can still enjoy Friday-night pizzas on the 30-Minutes-A-Day Eating Plan. For guilt-free, heart-smart versions, try these.

At a restaurant: Ask for half the cheese, double the sauce, and all the veggie toppings on a thin crust.

At home: Create individual gourmet pizzas by topping whole wheat pitas with sauce, precooked veggies (use up leftovers!), fresh basil, oregano, crushed black pepper, minced garlic, and fresh tomatoes. Add part-skim mozzarella or cut fat further by using grated Parmesan.

4. I Can't Believe It's Beans!

- *Three-bean salad:* Mix ½ cup each canned black beans and kidney beans (drained and rinsed), ½ cup thawed frozen string beans, and ¼ cup chopped yellow bell pepper and ¼ cup chopped green onions; toss with dressing made with 2 tsp olive oil, 2 tsp lemon juice or vinegar, ¼ tsp salt, ½ tsp chopped garlic, and your favorite herbs, and serve with ½ cup cold whole wheat noodles on a bed of spinach leaves.
- Mixed *salad greens* (rinse bagged greens) with 1 Tbsp olive oil dressing
- *Whole grain roll* or 1 slice whole grain bread

5. Seafood with Attitude

- Your choice of...
  Grilled or broiled 4-ounce piece of *salmon* brushed with olive oil and teriyaki sauce (from the ethnic foods aisle)
  or...

Mediterranean Baked Fish (recipe on page 236)

or...

Fish Baked on a Bed of Broccoli, Corn and Red Pepper (recipe on page 234)

or...

Shrimp Jambalaya (recipe on page 234)

- Steamed broccoli
- Cherry tomatoes with olive oil dressing

6. Meat Loaf Tonight

- Your choice of...
  Your favorite meat loaf recipe made with *lean ground beef*, 4-ounce serving

  or...

  Spinach-Stuffed Meat Loaf (recipe on page 239)

- *Oven Fries* (recipe on page 232) or baked sweet potato
- *Skillet Vegetable Side Dish* (recipe on page 233) or steamed precut veggie mix

7. Pasta Pleasures

- 1 cup *whole wheat spaghetti or pasta shapes* tossed with your choice of...

  - 1 cup scallops sautéed in 1 Tbsp olive oil, 1 tsp chopped garlic, lemon juice, and herbs to taste

  or...

  - 1 cup of your favorite jarred tomato sauce (no meat or cheese) mixed with ½ cup canned kidney or black beans (drained and rinsed)

Slash Your LDLs with Food

The smart food choices in the 30-Minutes-A-Day Eating Plan can dramatically lower your cholesterol naturally. This strategy could help you avoid medication or, if you must take a cholesterol-lowering drug, help you need a lower dose. Here are the reductions that top heart researchers think are possible if you take three key steps: Cut way back on saturated fat, get lots of soluble fiber (from oatmeal, barley, and at least two soluble fiber supplements per day), and have three servings of cholesterol-lowering margarine a day.

NEW EATING HABIT	POTENTIAL DROP IN LDLS
Cut saturated fat	Up to 12 points
Add 10 to 25 grams of soluble fiber	Up to 8 points
Add cholesterol-lowering margarine	Up to 16 points
Total drop	Up to 36 points

or...

- ½ cup canned or leftover cooked salmon, 2 tsp olive oil, 1 tsp chopped garlic, chopped red bell pepper, and herbs

  or...

- Meat sauce made by mixing 4 ounces sautéed lean ground beef or ground skinless chicken or turkey with jarred tomato sauce

- Mixed field greens (rinse bagged greens) with olive oil dressing

DESSERTS

Here are nine for that special occasion, each under 200 calories a serving.

- 1 cup *strawberries* (fresh or frozen, no added sugar) topped with $\frac{1}{2}$ cup low-fat *vanilla ice cream or frozen yogurt*

- *Homemade peach soft-serve:* In a blender or food processor, combine 1 cup frozen peaches, $\frac{1}{2}$ to 1 cup fat-free milk, and artificial sweetener to taste; process until smooth but not soupy.

- *Cinnamon baked apple:* Core 1 apple (Granny Smith works well) and loosely fill the center with cinnamon, raisins, nuts, and $\frac{1}{2}$ tsp brown sugar. Place 2 Tbsp water in the bottom of a microwaveable bowl and add the apple; cover and microwave 5 minutes, or until soft.

- Fresh or gently thawed frozen *raspberries* topped with 1 Tbsp *chocolate syrup* or 1 oz melted dark chocolate

- *Mixed fruit* (fresh; frozen; or juice packed, drained) topped with a sprinkle of coconut, chopped nuts, cinnamon, and $\frac{1}{2}$ tsp brown sugar

- *Walnut Raisin Pudding* (recipe on page 244)

- *Apricot and Pear Compote* (recipe on page 245)

- *Peach Cobbler* (recipe on page 245)

- *Raspberry Dessert Sauce with Cantaloupe* (recipe on page 246)

BEVERAGES

What you sip is just as important as what you eat. Fill your cup with these for a healthy heart.

- *Water.* Drink eight glasses a day. Research shows that drinking water cuts heart disease risk, possibly by diluting blood so it's less likely to clot.

- *Green and black tea.* Have one to three cups a day. Antioxidants in tea cut levels of LDLs and make arteries more flexible.

- *Red wine.* Women can have one 4-ounce glass per day; men can have up to two glasses. Red wine contains a heart-protecting antioxidant called resveratrol.

- *Cocoa.* Chocolate has antioxidants, too. Choose plain cocoa and make your own hot chocolate, or have an ounce of rich, dark chocolate candy.

What to avoid. Sodas, energy drinks, sweetened fruit juices, frothy coffee drinks (if you must have latte, ask for fat-free milk), sweetened iced tea, and beer.

Losing Weight the 30-Minutes-A-Day Way

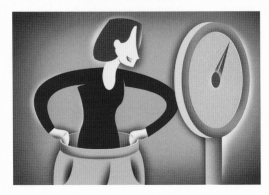

Weight loss begins with a deceptively simple formula, one that no fad diet, best-selling book, or renegade doctor can disprove: To lose weight, you must burn more calories in a day than you eat. Of course, if it were really that simple, 6 in 10 of us wouldn't be overweight. Stress, food

here are two key basics of eating for weight loss.

1. Get to Know What You Need

How many calories do you need to eat in a typical day? When we asked several hundred people that question in a survey, only 1 out of 5 said they knew the answer. However, pretty much everyone knew their weight, and nearly 9 in 10 said they knew their blood pressure numbers. That says a lot about our approach to health, doesn't it? After all, if you knew more precisely how much food you need to eat in a day, you probably wouldn't need to worry about those other numbers. So let's start by helping you figure out how many calories your body needs each day.

If you're inactive: You need about 13 calories per pound of body weight. For a 150-pound woman, that's 1,950 calories a day. For a 175-pound man, it's 2,275.

If you're slightly active (less than three exercise sessions per week, but regularly on your feet and moving): You need 14 calories

cravings, fatigue, temptation, office parties, happy hour, and lack of time contribute to weight gain—and make shedding pounds a challenge.

By following the 30-Minutes-A-Day Eating Plan as well as the advice in the rest of this book, you'll not only eat the right-size portions and get the calorie-burning exercise your

body needs, you'll also have the tools—such as ways to relax, feel happy, and reach out to friends—that help real change take place. This is an important point: Successful, lasting weight loss is rarely achieved from a diet plan alone. Rather, it requires a gradual shift to healthy living in all its forms. But to start, per pound to maintain your weight. For a 150-pound woman, that's 2,100 calories, and for a 175-pound man, 2,450.

If you're active (getting 30 to 60 minutes of exercise at least three times weekly): You need about 15 calories per pound of body weight. For a 150-pound woman, that's 2,250 calories; for a 175-pound man, it's 2,625.

To lose 1/2 pound a week—a realistic, achievable goal for people committing to small healthy lifestyle changes—you need 250 calories less per day. It's easy to eat 125 fewer calories; for example, have fruit instead of ice cream for dessert or pick a small hamburger instead of a large cheeseburger. It's just as easy to add 125 calories' worth of exercise with a 15-minute stroll at lunch and another after dinner.

2. Forget About Calorie Counting

Tallying calories can make you crazy. Even worse is trying to count grams of fat or grams of carbs or trying to keep score of the foods you eat, as so many diet plans have you do. You're smarter than they want you to think, so do what your common sense tells you: Eat a little less and move a little more. Do that every day,

and you *will* lose weight. For steady, healthy weight loss that lasts, there's no better way. In addition, the foods that are best for a healthy heart are exactly the foods you want to eat most for a healthy weight. Here's how to make the shift to lifelong healthy eating.

Let portions be your guide. Using the portion-control suggestions in "Right-Size Your Meals" on page 95, keep track of serving sizes. Expect some surprises: You may be eating more fruits and veggies than you realized (that's good), but you may also be underestimating the true quantity of breakfast cereal, pasta, ice cream, or snack foods, such as pretzels, you're eating. The consequence: You're eating more calories than you knew.

Start the day with breakfast. Skipping a morning meal leaves you so hungry that you can justify eating anything later on. Weight-loss winners in the National Weight Loss Control Registry—people who'd lost at least 30 pounds and kept it off—tended to eat in the morning.

Show up for lunch and dinner, too. The primary cause of nighttime binges is not eating enough during the day.

Eat in order. Finish off the "skinniest" parts of your meal first—salad, veggies, and

broth-based soups. Have meats and starches last so you'll be content with a little less.

Drink water, unsweetened tea, or diet drinks. Cutting out one 20-ounce sweetened drink per day—whether it's soda, sweetened tea, or lemonade—could help you lose 25 pounds in a year.

Keep a food journal for a week. It will show you what you're really eating and help you spot the times of day when you're skimping or overdoing it.

Don't be an island. Join a weight-loss support group online, at your church, or in your community. Plenty of research shows that dieting with a buddy helps both of you stick with the program, especially in the tough first month.

Don't eat merely out of boredom, stress, or habit. It's amazing how much we do this without even knowing it. We nibble while we watch TV or a movie; while we sit at the computer; when we need a break; or because it's 4 p.m., when we always walk to the vending machine for a candy bar. None of that eating is due to hunger—it's just habit. Find healthier ways to take breaks or deal with the stresses of everyday life. The best choice: a short walk followed by a glass of ice-cold water or a cup of hot tea.

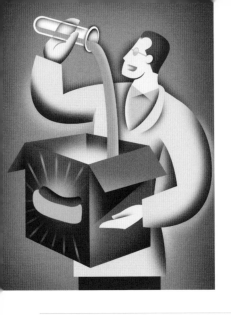

It's All in the Processing

GRAB THE BROCCOLI with cheese sauce from the freezer, the box of instant rice pilaf from the pantry, and the hot dogs from your fridge and squint at the fine print in the ingredient lists. You'll find lots of food additives in every one.

Repeat the experiment with any packaged food in the supermarket—and many in the health food store as well. Nearly all contain *something* that wasn't part of Mother Nature's original package. Safe? In the short term, yes—although some people have allergic reactions to some additives. Healthy? Compared with the foods our bodies were built to eat, definitely not.

No one likes to admit that he eats lots of food filled with additives and artificial flavorings, but in fact, processed, packaged foods have almost completely taken over the diet of Americans. In fact, nearly 90 percent

of our household food budgets are spent on processed foods, according to industry estimates. That doesn't leave a whole lot of money for fresh fruit, vegetables, seafood, lean meats, dairy, grains, or bread, does it?

Indeed, processed foods are the opposite of fresh. The majority are concocted in tasting labs by "food chemists," designed for maximum shelf life as well as maximum impact when put in your mouth. They are then manufactured on complex assembly lines in factory settings. To create the taste impact that keeps you buying more, processed foods are laden with sweeteners, salts, artificial flavors, factory-created fats, colorings, chemicals that alter texture, and preservatives. Then they are beautifully packaged and extensively marketed on television, in magazines, and in newspaper coupon supplements, as well as at the stores themselves. They are a very profitable business.

The trouble with processed foods isn't just what's added to them to make them so tasty; it's also what's been removed from them. Processed foods are often stripped of nutrients designed by nature to protect your heart, such as soluble fiber, antioxidants, and "good" fats. Combine that with additives known to endanger your cardiovascular system, particularly sugar, sodium, and trans fatty acids, and you can begin to see why a diet made up primarily of processed foods is a path to heart-health disaster.

A major tenet of the 30-Minutes-A-Day Plan is to put whole, natural, "outside the box" foods back on your plate, but without requiring you to spend hours shopping, chopping, or cooking. Much of the advice in the following chapters is geared to exactly that.

We realize that achieving this kind of diet is harder than it sounds. We are all used to eating food out of boxes, bags, and cans. That's what we grew up on and what stores are filled with. Plus, processed food manufacturers are smart—they make their products as convenient, simple, and cheap as possible to get us to buy them.

But the health case against them is strong, and for you to achieve your heart-health goals, you need to take them seriously. In this chapter, we'll explain more about the processing of foods and highlight the four ingredients you should focus on first and foremost and purge from your diet. Then, in the chapters ahead, we'll detail the foods you should eat most and provide tips and recipes to make it as easy as possible to do so.

Inside the Food Factory

How do you know if a food has been processed? A general signal is that it arrived at the store in a ready-for-sale,

The Health Robbers: 10 Ways Processing *Hurts* Your Food

Most of the foods we eat are no longer in a natural state. Fish comes from "factory farms" instead of from algae-rich wild waters, beef cattle are grain fed instead of naturally grass fed, most eggs come from corn-fed chickens instead of those that munch on field greens, and fruits and veggies are robbed of their fiber and nutrients. To make matters worse, they're injected with unhealthy doses of salt, sugar, and/or "bad fats" when they become potato chips, canned soup, fruit drinks, and more. Here's how modern technology makes food *less* healthy.

- It adds heart-threatening trans fats and saturated fats.
- It adds blood pressure–raising sodium.
- It adds blood sugar–elevating sweeteners.
- It removes natural fiber.
- It removes vitamins, minerals, and antioxidants.
- It adds chemical preservatives, flavors, and colors.

- It adds antibiotics and growth hormones to meat and dairy products.
- It raises the risk of contamination by bacteria, viruses, and parasites.
- It replaces good omega-3 fatty acids in meat and fish with inflammation-promoting omega-6 fatty acids.
- It replaces naturally balanced nutrients with a more limited range of man-made vitamins and minerals in fortified foods.

sealed package in a form different from its original, natural state. That would describe most canned, frozen, dehydrated, bottled, or boxed food items. We're talking about cereal, ice cream, soup, frozen pizza, candy, jarred spaghetti sauce, pretzels, and almost everything found in the central aisles of the supermarket.

Of course, not all prepackaged foods are problematic. Milk, yogurt, and cheese all arrive at the store in their final packaging after some type of pasteurizing process, and some very healthy organic spaghetti sauces and energy bars have few if any unnatural ingredients. The problem is mostly with foods that have been dramatically altered for convenience, taste, or long shelf life. These are the foods with lengthy ingredient lists that include chemicals the typical person has never heard of.

Among the additives we typically consume each day are artificial flavorings developed by chemists from nonfood sources; food dyes, such as yellow #6 and red #40 (the most widely used food coloring in the United States); butylated hydroxyanisole to keep fats and oils from going rancid; thickeners such as carageenan; sulfite preservatives; phosphoric acid to give cola drinks their tang; sweeteners to heighten taste; and synthetic vitamins and minerals—replacements for nutrients lost to processing.

Vitamins in a Bowl: Are Fortified Foods Nutritious?

Everyday foods with pumped-up nutritional profiles—breakfast cereal with 100 percent of eight essential vitamins and minerals, orange juice with bone-building calcium, milk with added vitamin D, bread with folic acid—*look* like health superstars, but do you need them?

The answer: yes and no. While fortified and enriched foods may help fill nutritional gaps, such as bringing a pregnant woman's intake of folic acid up to par to protect her baby from birth defects, they aren't better than a healthy, balanced diet, nutrition experts maintain. (In the United States, food fortification began in the 1920s with the addition of iodine to table salt to prevent goiter.) Here's what you need to know.

- Fortified foods should still be nutritious in their own right. Look for natural nutrients first and consider fortification a bonus. Choose calcium-rich low-fat milk (it will be fortified with vitamins A and D to help your body absorb calcium); naturally vitamin C–packed, 100 percent orange juice fortified with calcium; and whole grain, high-fiber breakfast cereals (if they've got added nutrients, it's a plus.) A little extra nutrition is fine, but it shouldn't be the reason to choose a food.

- If you take a daily multivitamin (and most of us should), you don't need a day's worth of vitamins added to your food as well. You *do* need fiber, good fats, and the hundreds of protective phytochemicals in fruits and veggies—many of which have yet to be discovered.

- Don't bother with mood-elevating, brain-enhancing, immune-boosting herbal add-ons. Soup with depression-lifting St. John's wort? Fruit juice with cold-fighting echinacea? Skip 'em. You're better off taking herbs separately, in expert-recommended doses.

In all, American food manufacturers mix 3,000 different additives into our foods. Some aren't even on the labels. For example, some fruits lose their vivid flavors during processing as juice, so manufacturers mix missing flavor ingredients back in, and some artificial flavors (which may be listed simply as "artificial flavor") contain dozens of chemicals—top-secret formulas devised, most often, at a string of chemical companies arrayed along the New Jersey Turnpike.

Are They Safe?

The truth is, many additives have not undergone safety testing—they're in a category that the FDA calls "generally recognized as safe" because they've been used for decades without causing apparent trouble. (Newly developed additives, however, need to meet specific safety standards.) The rest of the story? Food-safety advocates such as the Center for Science in the Public Interest (CSPI) still consider some additives risky because they cause allergic or asthmatic reactions, headaches, and other health problems in some people, and some food colorings, CSPI claims, may cause cancer in lab animals.

Chemicals aside, food processing often entails stripping down natural foods to their components before creating the final product. As you'll see in a moment, when whole grains are refined this way, the healthiest part of the grain is often left behind. This is often true even in seemingly innocuous processes. For example, a whole orange has much more fiber than a cup of freshly squeezed orange juice, so even this simple, natural "processing" reduces the healthfulness of the original, natural food.

It would be nearly impossible today to eat a diet devoid of chemicals and untouched by modern processing methods. It is possible, however, to reduce your consumption of the additives and refinements known to cause the most damage to your health and heart. Here, then, are the big four. Focus your efforts on these, and you'll take a major step toward protecting your heart.

1 TRANS FATS: A Man-Made Disaster

Trans fats are the phantom fats lurking in moist bakery muffins and crispy crackers, microwave popcorn and fast-food French fries, and even in the stick margarine you may rely on as a "heart-healthy" alternative to saturated-fat-laden butter.

Once hailed as a cheap, heart-friendly replacement for butter, lard, and coconut oil in processed foods, trans fats were recently denounced by one Harvard nutrition expert as "the biggest food-processing disaster in U.S. history." Why? Research now reveals that trans fats are twice as dangerous for your heart as saturated fat and cause an estimated 30,000 to 100,000 premature deaths from heart disease each year!

The trouble is, they're everywhere—in cookies, crackers, icing, potato chips, snack foods, margarine, doughnuts, and muffins, plus commercially prepared French fries, onion rings, and fried chicken and fish. Here's what you need to know about escaping the trans fat trap.

Trans Fats: *The Details*

✓ **Processed poison.** Trans fats are produced when liquid vegetable oil is heated and transformed into a solid form called partially hydrogenated oil. The process was first discovered a century ago; today, trans fats are found in 42,000 different food products. They keep stick margarine and vegetable shortening solid at room temperature, keep baked goods moist and snack foods crunchy, and extend the shelf life of many foods. In the 1980s and 1990s, fast-food chains filled their fryers with partially hydrogenated oil instead of beef fat, citing heart-healthy benefits. Food makers introduced products containing "no saturated fat" that were instead loaded with these bad fats.

✓ **How trans fats attack your heart.** Trans fats are *worse* for your heart than saturated fats because they boost levels of "bad" LDL cholesterol *and* decrease "good" HDL cholesterol. And unlike sat fats, trans fats also raise levels of artery-clogged lipoprotein(a) and triglycerides. Some researchers also suspect that trans fats further threaten your heart by increasing inflammation and making cells resistant to insulin.

✓ **Label detective.** Trans fats will be listed on the Nutrition Facts panel on foods beginning in 2006. Until then, check the ingredient list for any of these terms: "partially hydrogenated," "fractionated" or "hydrogenated" (fully hydrogenated fats are not a heart threat, but some trans fats are mislabeled as "hydrogenated"). The higher up partially hydrogenated oil is in the list, the more trans fat the product contains.

Also, don't automatically trust claims such as "zero grams of trans fat." Products with less than 0.5 gram per serving are allowed to list trans fat content as zero. Eat a few servings, and you rack up a lot.

✓ **Safe upper limit.** None. The Institute of Medicine suggests cutting trans fats out of your diet as much as possible.

✓ **Avoid trans fats for this heart bonus.** Replacing trans fats with good fats could cut your heart attack risk by a whopping 53 percent.

8 Ways to Escape the Trans Fat Trap

1. Choose tub margarine instead of stick margarine, and look for brands with the lowest trans fat content.

2. Use olive oil instead of stick margarine for sautéing.

3. Sprinkle slivered nuts or sunflower seeds on salads instead of bacon bits.

4. Snack on a small handful of nuts or a box of raisins rather than potato chips or processed crackers. Or try peanut butter or other nut-butter spreads (nonhydrogenated) on celery, bananas, or rice or popcorn cakes.

5. Shop the perimeter of the store. Most processed foods, which contain a lot of trans fats, are on the inner aisles of the supermarket.

6. When you do purchase processed foods, choose lower-fat versions of crackers, cereals, and desserts.

7. Skip fast-food fries. Get a side salad, a plain baked potato, or, for the kids, a healthy alternative such as sliced fruit (now becoming available at more fast-food chains).

8. When you have time, make your own pancakes, waffles, and muffins instead of using store-bought versions or a trans fat–packed mix. Make extra and freeze some. (See Heart Healthy Recipes on page 228 for recipes for Oatmeal Waffles, Apple-Topped Oatcakes, and Hearty Carrot Muffins.)

2 REFINED CARBS: Stripped of Their Goodness

If you "accessorize" your meals with white bread, rolls, sugary cereal, white rice, or white pasta, you're not alone. Most, if not all, of the six to seven helpings of grains most of us eat every day are refined; less than one is an unrefined, heart-loving whole grain.

Choosing refined over whole grains boosts your heart attack risk by up to 30 percent, so you've got to be a savvy shopper: You may think you're eating healthy whole grains when in fact that brown bread or "multigrain" cereal on your table is an impostor. Don't be fooled by deceptive label claims such as "made with wheat flour" or "seven grain," or by white-flour breads topped with a sprinkling of oats or colored brown with molasses. Often, they're just the same old refined stuff that raises the risk of high cholesterol, high blood pressure, heart attacks, insulin resistance, diabetes, and belly fat.

A 21st-century malady? Not really. In ancient Egypt, rich folks feasted on breads made from hand-sieved grain. In European manor houses, the kitchen staff filtered wheat flour through silken sieves to remove those pesky (and actually nutrition rich) brown bits. Here's what we know today.

Refined Carbs: The Details

✓ **Processed poison.** Nobody's sifting wheat grains through silk these days. Grains are now commercially milled and polished—in fact, a 60-pound bushel of wheat leaves the mill as 43 pounds of white flour. What's left behind? Wheat bran—the brown, fiber-rich outer layer of the wheat grain, filled with niacin, thiamin, riboflavin, magnesium, phosphorus, iron, and zinc—along with wheat germ, the grain's nutrient and fat-rich inner layer, a concentrated source of niacin, thiamin, riboflavin, vitamin E, magnesium, phosphorus, iron, and zinc, plus some protein and fat. Together, the bran and germ contain up to 90 percent of the grain's nutrients. Refining's benefit for producers: longer shelf life.

✓ **How refined grains attack your heart.** At least seven major studies show that women and men who eat more whole grains (including dark bread, whole grain breakfast cereals, popcorn, cooked oatmeal, brown rice, bran, and other grains, such as bulgur and kasha) have 20 to 30 percent less heart disease. In contrast, those who opt for

6 Ways to Go Whole Grain

Aim for three servings of whole grains per day. Here's how to swap refined grains for the good stuff.

1. Switch to a high-fiber cereal such as oatmeal, Cheerios, Raisin Bran, Total, Wheaties, Spoon-Size Shredded Wheat, or Grape-Nuts.
2. Substitute whole wheat toast for bagels and low-fat multigrain muffins in place of pastries.
3. Make sandwiches with whole grain breads or rolls.
4. Expand your grain repertoire with whole grains such as kasha, brown rice, wild rice, bulgur, and whole wheat tortillas.
5. Use wild rice or barley in soups, stews, casseroles, and salads.
6. Add whole grains, such as cooked brown rice, or whole grain bread crumbs to ground meat or poultry for extra body.

refined grains have more heart attacks, insulin resistance, and high blood pressure. Why? Blood sugar levels climb higher and faster after you eat a slice of white bread or a scoop of white rice than if you opt for whole wheat bread or brown rice. This raises insulin levels, which in turn decreases levels of "good" HDLs, jacks up risky triglycerides, raises blood pressure, and prompts blood to clot more easily. It also raises your risk of insulin resistance and type 2 diabetes.

That's not all. When Tufts University nutritionists measured the waistlines of 459 people, they found that those who ate the most refined grains saw their midsections expand by ½ inch per year. Belly fat pumps out heart-threatening hormones and fatty acids 24/7. A "white" diet also deprives your arteries of a huge range of protective substances found in whole grains, including cholesterol-lowering soluble fiber and antioxidants that shield LDL cholesterol from the damage that leads to artery-clogging plaque.

✓ **Safe upper limit**. As little as possible. Go for at least three whole grain servings a day at first.

✓ **Label detective.** Read the ingredient list on packaged grain products; the first ingredient should be whole wheat or another whole grain, such as oats, and the fiber content should be at least 3 grams per serving.

✓ **Avoid refined grains for this heart bonus.** Simply choosing whole grains instead of the refined type could cut your risk of heart attack by 30 percent and reduce your risk of metabolic syndrome by 33 percent.

3 SALT: Extra Flavor, Extra Trouble

Here's a mystery: You shake a few grains of salt on your scrambled eggs, add a pinch to your mixed green salad at lunch, and then scatter a bit more on dinner's baked potato and roasted chicken. The total? Scarcely ½ teaspoon. Yet somehow, most of us actually consume nearly 2 heaping teaspoons of blood pressure–raising sodium chloride daily. Where does it all come from?

Three-quarters of the sodium in our diets *isn't* from your saltshaker. It's hidden in processed foods, such as canned veggies and canned soups; condiments, such as soy sauce and Worcestershire sauce; fast-food burgers (and fries, of course); and cured or preserved meats, such as bacon, ham, and deli turkey.

Sure, some sodium occurs naturally in unprocessed edibles, including milk, beets, celery, and even some drinking water. And that's a good thing: Sodium is necessary for life. It helps regulate blood pressure, maintains the body's fluid balance, transmits nerve impulses, makes muscles—including your heart—contract, and keeps your senses of taste, smell, and touch working properly.

You need a little every day to replace what's lost to sweat, tears, and other excretions. But is more salt dangerous? Scientists—and the salt industry—have vigorously debated this for decades. Just recently, the verdict was handed down by an impartial government panel called the Institute of Medicine: More salt *is* bad for your heart.

Salt: *The Details*

✓ **Processed poison.** Since prehistoric times, humans have used salt as a food. Today, food processors dump nearly 4.2 million tons per year into processed foods, for many reasons. It improves the texture of cheese, helps preserve and moisturize meats, keeps fats evenly distributed in sausage, and makes yeast breads more tender. No wonder it's in everything from bread to breakfast cereal, canned goods to fast foods, and butter to margarine.

✓ **How salt attacks your heart.** Your body needs a precise concentration of sodium; eating extra salt prompts it to retain fluid simply to dilute the extra sodium in your bloodstream. This raises blood volume, which forces your heart to work harder; at the same time, it makes veins and arteries constrict. The combination raises blood pressure.

Does it raise blood pressure for everyone, or are just a few unlucky folks stuck with salt sensitivity? That issue has been hotly debated for decades. The truth is, while 30 to 60 percent of people with high blood pressure and 25 to 50 percent of people with normal blood pressure can lower their pressures by cutting back on salt, some researchers believe that nearly everyone could cut their blood pressure at least a little bit by reining in the chips, pretzels, and automatic salt sprinkling at meals. An even better plan: Eat less salt and more of the produce, dairy foods, and whole grains that provide pressure-lowering minerals such as potassium and calcium. Often, people with hypertension are low in these minerals.

✓ **Safe upper limit.** 1,500 milligrams of sodium per day, about the amount in 3/4 teaspoon of salt. (Table salt, by the way, is 40 percent sodium and 60 percent chloride.) Older people should eat even less to counteract the natural rise in blood pressure that comes with age. People over 50 should strive

8 Ways to Shake the Salt Habit

You're not really addicted to salt. Try these salt-reduction strategies, and within a week or two, you won't miss it at all.

1. Omit salt from recipes or automatically reduce sodium by 25 percent by measuring out the same amount of kosher or coarse salt instead—the coarse granules of these salts don't pack as tightly into a measuring spoon.

2. Take the shaker off your kitchen table or switch to light salt (50 percent less sodium) or a salt substitute, which uses a stand-in such as potassium chloride.

3. Shake an alternative seasoning. Try a spice blend, such as Mrs. Dash, or go with a squirt of lemon, some crushed garlic (*not* garlic salt!), or thyme.

4. Choose canned foods with little or no added sodium.

5. Choose processed foods (such as frozen entrées) with less than 5 percent of the Daily Value for sodium in each serving.

6. Give unsalted or reduced-sodium pretzels, chips, and condiments a try.

7. When buying low-fat cheese, go for a low-sodium variety.

8. Read over-the-counter drug labels (yes, they have Nutrition Facts labels, too). Some items, especially antacids, can be high in sodium. Ask the pharmacist about lower-sodium options.

for 1,300 milligrams; those over 70 should aim for 1,200 milligrams. In reality, most of us eat about 4,000 milligrams per day.

✓ **Avoid excess salt for this heart bonus.** Reducing your sodium intake by just 300 milligrams (the amount in about two slices of cheese) cuts systolic pressure (the first number in a blood pressure reading) by 2 to 4 points and reduces diastolic pressure (the second number) by 1 to 2 points. Cut more, and pressure drops even lower.

4 HIGH-FRUCTOSE CORN SYRUP: Liquid Sweetness

America is a country drowning in sweetness. In fact, the amount of processed sugar we eat and drink every year has soared nearly 30 percent since 1983. Although the USDA recommends we get no more than the equivalent of 10 teaspoons of sugar a day, the average American downs about 34 teaspoons—more than three times as much.

When you ask most people what makes food sweet, they'll usually say plain old sugar. But since 1970, a quiet coup d'état has been taking place inside your favorite snack cakes, ice cream, and sodas. Indeed, honey or cane and beet sugar once sweetened most of these; today, corn syrups rule the roost—and their reach extends far beyond sweet treats.

It's easy to see why: Compared to traditional sweeteners, high-fructose corn syrup costs less to make, is sweeter to the taste, and mixes more easily with other ingredients. Today, we down nearly 63 pounds of it per person per year in drinks and sweets as well as in bread, beer, bacon, spaghetti sauce, and even ketchup.

But high-fructose corn syrup may not be so sweet. Many nutritionists believe it's a major culprit in America's obesity epidemic. What's more, research is beginning to suggest that the chemical structure of the fructose in this liquid sweetener may wreak havoc with human metabolism, raising the risk of heart disease and diabetes.

High-Fructose Corn Syrup: The Details

✓ **Processed poison**. In the early 1970s, Japanese food researchers hit upon a way to turn cornstarch into thick, sweet syrup that's 55 percent fructose and 45 percent glucose. Between 1970 and 1990, U.S. consumption of corn syrup increased 1,000 percent, for some unexpected reasons.

High-fructose corn syrup can stop freezer burn, so it's in many frozen foods; it gives bread an inviting brown color and soft texture, so it's also in whole wheat bread, hamburger buns, and even English muffins. By the year 2000, it was the sole source of sugar in soft drinks in the United States.

✓ **How high-fructose corn syrup attacks your heart.** This sugar revolution may be fueling America's obesity epidemic. While opponents claim the problem is simply due to out-of-control portions, researchers say high-fructose corn syrup's chemical structure *encourages* overeating by disrupting three key appetite-controlling hormones.

Unlike traditional sugars, the new corn syrup doesn't turn on appetite-suppressing insulin and leptin. Research from the University of California, Davis, also reveals that fructose doesn't suppress ghrelin, a hormone that *increases* hunger and appetite. The result: Instead of putting the brakes on appetite, high-fructose corn syrup pushes the accelerator. It also seems to force the liver to pump more heart-threatening triglycerides into the bloodstream, and it may zap your body's reserves of chromium, a mineral important for healthy levels of cholesterol, insulin, and blood sugar.

✓ **Safe upper limit.** The USDA recommends limiting added sugar—everything from the stuff sweetening your yogurt to the sugar you spoon into your morning coffee—to 10 to 12 teaspoons a day. The reality: Most Americans consume about 31 teaspoons' worth each day.

✓ **Label detective.** Beyond high-fructose corn syrup, look for "corn sweetener," "corn syrup," or "corn syrup solids" on the ingredient list.

✓ **Avoid high-fructose corn syrup for this heart bonus.** Lower blood sugar, insulin, and triglycerides. Cutting out corn syrups may also make weight loss easier.

No More High-Fructose Corn Syrup

Here are four ways to whisk this dangerous sweetener out of your diet.

1. Enjoy natural sweets. We're talking about fruit—fresh, frozen (without syrup), canned in its own juice, or dried (provided it's not sugar coated). Yes, fruit contains fructose, but in smaller quantities than in high-fructose corn syrup. Plus, fruit brings you a wealth of fiber, vitamins, and minerals and a host of antioxidants.

2. Limit "liquid candy"—that's soda, processed fruit juice, and sweetened iced tea. Switch to seltzer with a splash of orange or lemon juice; plain water; or, if you just love soda, a diet version.

3. Take your reading glasses to the supermarket. Even applesauce, stewed tomatoes, and pasta sauce may contain corn syrup—but usually, there's a syrup-free version right next to it on the shelf.

4. Rediscover (low-fat) milk. Milk consumption in the United States has dropped by 58 percent, and as a result, levels of calcium—a mineral important for maintaining healthy blood pressure—have dropped as well. Milk is an outstanding alternative to soda with meals.

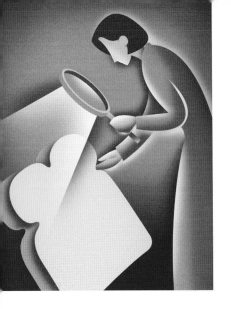

The Truth About Carbs

NET CARBS. IMPACT CARBS. Fit carbs. Smart carbs. The mania for restricted-carbohydrate eating programs has brought a whole new vocabulary to the world of nutrition, hundreds of competing diet plans and cookbooks to bookstores, and more than 900 new "low-carb" products to supermarket shelves in the past five years. Without question, this has stirred a major controversy among nutritionists, doctors, and the federal government.

Among the new offerings are cookbooks with recipes for indulgent low-carb desserts and low-carb slow-cooker dinners, a rescue manual for low-carbers who've fallen off the wagon, and even a book to help you choose the best low-carb diet book. On store shelves: low-carb breads and pastas, chocolate candy and creamy cheesecake, energy bars and crunchy pork rinds, beer, and even a reduced-carb substitute for fat-free milk. (We ask: Does anyone *need* a substitute for fat-free milk?)

Behind this giant craze is one central claim: faster, easier weight loss thanks to lower, steadier blood sugar. The reality: It's not nearly that simple. It *is* smart to cut *refined* carbs out of your diet—goodbye doughnuts and white bread, white rice and potato chips—but many plans pose an immediate threat to your heart by demonizing all carbs. Blacklisting fruit, veggies, and whole grains robs your cardiovascular system of the health protectors you need every day: soluble fiber, vitamins, minerals, and antioxidants. What's more, research shows that in the long run, a moderate-carb diet that includes these healthy foods may be as good as, or better than, a low-carb plan for keeping unwanted pounds off.

As for those high-priced, often odd-tasting low-carb foods, know this: A chocolate bar touting "2 net carbs" *sounds* skinny, but it probably has as many calories and as much fat as its normal-carb cousin. Low-carb is a marketing ploy as seductive as low-fat was in the 1990s. The promises on the products' wrappers make them seem healthier, leaner, almost magic—but a candy bar is still a candy bar, governed by nature's first rule of weight gain: Eat too many calories, and you will gain weight.

Low-Carb Myths and Truths

The premise of all low-carb foods and diet plans begins with nutrition-science basics. Carbohydrates *do* raise blood sugar, because they provide so much of your body's preferred source of fuel: glucose. When glucose levels rise, your pancreas releases a flood of insulin that prompts cells to store sugar. Advocates say that eating a diet low in carbs makes weight loss easier because low, steady blood sugar conquers food cravings. But the next step in the low-carb equation is open to debate: Proponents say these diets also change your metabolism so your body breaks down more fats, and—voilà—fewer of the calories you eat are stored as flab.

Low-carb weight-loss plans do work—for a while. Pounds drop quickly at first because burning stored carbs (called glycogen) releases water. Quite simply, you lose excess water weight. Nutritionists say, though, that low-carb weight loss isn't metabolic magic, just the working-out of nature's first rule of weight loss: Eat fewer calories, and you will shed pounds. Some low-carbers say this special way of eating eliminates cravings, but

Glycemic Index Tricks

The glycemic index ranks carbohydrates based on their effects on blood sugar levels. Carbs that break down quickly in the body have the highest GI ratings; carbs that release sugar gradually into the bloodstream are low on the GI index. Researchers say that eating low-GI foods can cut your risk of diabetes, heart disease, and even cancer.

The trouble is, the GI index is a rather strange list: Carrots have a higher GI than pound cake or doughnuts, for example. Also, computing a food's ultimate effect on blood sugar requires you to consider portion size, other foods eaten at the same meal (fat and protein slow sugar absorption), and how the food is prepared—for example, a slow-rising bread has a lower GI than one made with rapid-acting yeast.

Too complex? You bet. Even experts suggest that you forget the formula but keep the GI idea in mind by following this advice to lower the GI of any meal.

- Eat breakfast cereals based on oats, barley, and bran, as well as whole grain breads.

- Choose whole fruits rather than higher-GI juices.

- Eat lots of veggies.

- Choose vinaigrette dressing for salad. Researchers have found that vinegar reduces a meal's glycemic index significantly.

- Have some fat and protein. Snacking on baby carrots or an apple? Add a dab of peanut butter.

others feel headachy and nauseated. Burning fat without carbohydrates produces substances called ketones, which can decrease appetite, but there's a danger because sustained high ketone levels may deplete mineral stores in bones, leaving them fragile. Here's the rest of the low-carb story.

LOW-CARB DIETS DON'T GO THE DISTANCE FOR WEIGHT LOSS

Carb-conscious eating may speed up early weight loss, but not much more. In a year-long study of 63 dieters, University of Pennsylvania researchers found that low-carb dieters dropped 4 percent more weight than those following a conventional low-cal plan in the first six months—but both groups achieved nearly identical weight losses after one year.

When researchers at the National Weight Control Registry looked at the diets of 2,681 successful dieters who had maintained at least a 30-pound weight loss for a year or more, they expected to see many low-carb diet adherents. They were shocked to find just 25, or 1 percent of the total group. Their conclusion: Low-carb plans didn't produce a lasting metabolic change that kept pounds off.

The New Carb Glossary

To help reduce that spinning feeling in your head from reading so many conflicting reports on carbohydrates, here are the terms you need to know.

Carbohydrates. One of the three main forms of food that make up the human diet (the other two are fats and protein). More precisely, carbohydrates are a wide range of organic compounds, created by plants, that include carbon, hydrogen, and oxygen. Starches and sugars are among the carbohydrates we eat.

Carbs. A shorthand version of *carbohydrates*. The health community uses the term merely because it's easier to say than the full four-syllable word.

Complex carbs. Carbohydrates with a more intricate chemical composition, which require more time to break down into basic sugars during digestion. Plant-based foods in their raw or natural form are mostly composed of complex carbs, as well as fiber, plant-based fats, and healing nutrients. It is this winning combination of nutritious ingredients and slow digestion that makes plants in their natural form among the healthiest foods available to us humans.

Simple carbs. These carbs are chemically simple, so they digest quickly into glucose, or blood sugar. While some plant foods—such as potatoes and carrots—contain lots of simple carbohydrates, most of the simple carbs in our diet are a result of refining done at food factories. White flour, refined sugar, and white rice are the most common simple carbohydrates. The process that simplifies carbohydrates often removes the fiber, plant fats, and micronutrients from the original plant, thus stripping it of much of its nutrition value.

Good carbs. What many diet experts call complex carbs.

Bad carbs. What many diet experts call simple carbs.

Net carbs (also known as smart carbs or impact carbs). A recently fabricated concept; essentially, net carbs are complex carbs minus their fiber and certain natural sweeteners. The theory is that net carbs are the parts of the carb that affect blood sugar levels. However, most nutritionists consider net-carb measurements to be gimmicky, invalid, and not useful. The FDA doesn't consider it a legitimate nutritional measurement and has set no standards for the term's use.

A HIGH-FAT, SUPER-LOW-CARB DIET THREATENS YOUR HEART

The Atkins Diet—the oldest and most famous of the low-carb regimens—allows a mere 20 grams of carbs per day in the earliest, strictest phase, putting most grains, beans, fruits, breads, rice, potatoes, pastas, and starchy vegetables off-limits. At the same time, it allows generous amounts of beef, pork, chicken, eggs, and butter.

Unlimited access to bacon cheeseburgers is tempting, but a low-carb diet that's essentially an all-you-can-eat saturated-fat buffet may increase your risk of heart attack and stroke, the American Heart Association cautions. All that sat fat can raise levels of heart-threatening LDL cholesterol—and at the same time shortchange you on the antioxidants from fruits, veggies, and grains that protect arteries from plaque formation. (Low-carb diets are also high in protein, which makes them risky for people with diabetes because they can speed the progression of diabetic kidney disease.)

LOW-CARB *ISN'T* LOW-CALORIE

Many low-carb products undermine weight-loss efforts because they're packed with as many—or even more—calories than "regular carb" versions. Many are also higher in fat. This is especially true of reduced-carb comfort foods such as ice cream, bread, pasta, and snack bars. A 1-ounce low-carb chocolate bar with 120 calories or a 270-calorie scoop of low-carb Rocky Road ice cream won't do your hips any favors.

"It's the calories, not the carbohydrates," notes Robert O. Bonow, M.D., former president of the American Heart Association. "America is gaining weight because people are eating more calories than they can burn and getting less exercise."

LOW-CARB JUNK FOOD IS STILL…JUNK

Indulging in a low-carb snack food with the belief that it's a better weight-loss choice than a piece of fruit, a serving of veggies, or a handful of whole grain crackers (trans fat–free, of course) puts you in double jeopardy: You've just robbed your body of a host of heart-healthy nutrients and fiber, and you may have eaten a ton of empty calories. Example: For 40 grams of carbs a day, you could eat ½ cup of lentils, a cup of carrots, an orange, and a slice of light seven-grain bread (total calories: 40; plus a hefty dose of antioxidants, vitamins, and minerals). Getting those 40 grams from low-carb snack foods could supply up to *1,440 calories* and very few nutrients.

Low-Carb Lessons

What about refined carbs—sweets, white bread, white rice, and white pasta? Here's where low-carb diets offer a big kernel of truth. These "bad" carbs have been linked to heart disease, diabetes, and even cancer. Here's why: Refined carbs make blood sugar levels spike quickly because they've been stripped of the good stuff that slows digestion, including fiber and bits of fat. As a result, your pancreas pumps out extra insulin to help cells absorb the extra sugar, and your body endures toxic insulin levels that wreak havoc with cholesterol and triglyceride levels.

Eating lots of refined carbs *doubled* heart risk in the landmark Nurses' Health Study. According to researcher Simin Liu,

M.D., Sc.D., of Brigham and Women's Hospital and Harvard Medical School in Boston, a diet high in refined carbs boosts triglycerides, suppresses levels of heart-helping HDL cholesterol, and may contribute to high blood pressure and artery-threatening inflammation. That's why the 30-Minutes-A-Day Plan will help you cut back on refined carbs.

Buried in the low-carb hype is a second truth: Eating fat and protein is important. Both keep blood sugar levels steady, thus cutting food cravings. "Good fats" won't raise your LDLs, keep HDLs from dropping (a danger on low-fat diets), and protect your heart against dangerous out-of-rhythm beats. Protein low in saturated fat, such as lean beef, chicken, or eggs, supplies heart-protecting nutrients and amino acids to rebuild heart muscle cells and other cells throughout your body. On the 30-Minutes-A-Day Plan, you'll find satisfying good fats and protein at every meal.

Smart Carbs, the 30-Minutes-A-Day Way

When it comes to carbs, our plan is firmly in the moderate camp. The fact is, good carbs—fruit, vegetables, and whole grains—are essential guardians of heart health. The proof: A University of Minnesota review of 10 studies involving 91,000 men and 245,000 women found that for every 10 grams of fiber from fruit that study volunteers ate every day, the risk of fatal heart disease dropped a staggering 30 percent. For every 10 grams of cereal fiber, risk dropped 15 percent.

That's not much food for a lot of protection: You'd get 10 grams of fiber in a day if you ate an apple, a pear, and two dried apricot halves. You'd get 10 grams of cereal fiber from a bowl of Kellogg's Raisin Bran and one slice of whole wheat toast. Vegetables count, too: A study at the Harvard School of Public Health found that for each additional serving of veggies you eat daily, heart risk drops 4 percent.

Fruits and vegetables are packed with heart helpers, including fiber to cut cholesterol and discourage blood clots; antioxidants; blood pressure–lowering potassium; and folate and vitamin B_6, key nutrients for lowering levels of homocysteine, an amino acid that can damage artery walls and prompt formation of dangerous blood clots.

Good carbs can also help you control your weight. As part of the Nurses' Health Study, researchers at the Harvard School of Public Health followed more than 74,000 women from 1984 to 1996. They found that women who consumed more whole grains consistently weighed less than women who consumed fewer. Why? Fiber-packed good carbs aid weight loss by keeping you full longer (they hold more water in your digestive system), slowing digestion down, and whisking some calories out of the body unabsorbed.

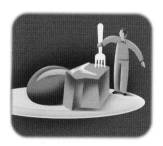

Overcoming
Portion Distortion

Signs of the super-size times: Restaurants have swapped their 10-inch plates, once the industry standard, for 12-inch versions. Why? More room for portions big enough to feed not just you, but the entire family—8 cups of spaghetti, a pound of ribs, or a mountain of 70 French fries.

We've super-sized in our own kitchens, too. When researchers at the University of North Carolina compared at-home portion sizes today with those of 30 years ago, they were shocked to discover that a serving of chips or pretzels is now 93 calories bigger, hamburgers now contain 93 more calories, and a serving of French fries is now up by 68 calories.

Portion distortion is one of the prime causes of America's obesity epidemic, yet most of us don't even realize that we overeat—or that when it comes to reining in calories, serving size is crucial. In fact, one recent survey found that 62 percent of Americans believe restaurant portions are *smaller* today than 10 years ago; 80 percent said the portions they eat at home are the same or smaller.

We're overlooking out-of-control portions for a variety of reasons, from seductive weight-loss myths to genetic programming to economics.

We think *what* we eat matters more than *how much* we eat. When the American Institute for Cancer Research surveyed Americans about their eating habits, a surprising 78 percent said that eating certain types of food while avoiding others was more central to their weight-management efforts than eating less food. The problem: We're missing the big picture—for weight control, it's total calories that count.

We're programmed to eat whatever is in front of us. When researchers at Pennsylvania State University served study volunteers one of two portions of macaroni and cheese—either a reasonable 2½ cups or a whopping 5 cups—the average volunteer ate 30 percent more food when given the bigger portion, without reporting feeling any fuller. "Men and women, normal-weight and overweight individuals, restrained and unrestrained eaters, all responded to larger portion size by eating more," notes portion-size expert Barbara Rolls, Ph.D., of Penn State's College of Health and Human Development.

We think more food is a better bargain. Plates piled high with pancakes or lasagna or that 20-ounce steak look impressive when the server sets them on your table. Eateries can afford to pile on large portions because food is one of the smaller-ticket items on their budgets (rent and staff salaries cost more)—but getting more for your money isn't good for your waistline or your health.

The result? The USDA estimates that Americans now consume 148 more calories per day than 20 years ago. That doesn't sound like much, but by itself, it works out to an extra 15 pounds every year. Couple that with a more sedentary lifestyle, and our troubles with weight make much more sense.

The bad news about big portions: When we overeat at one meal, we really don't cut back at the next. When researchers in Penn State's portion lab doubled the portions they fed a group of volunteers, women ate 530 more calories and men ate 803 more over the course of a day—even though they'd also overeaten on the previous day.

Perfect Portion Size Guide

Shocking news: Most of us underestimate portions, and calories, by at least 25 percent—meaning that you could eat hundreds of extra calories every day and not even know it. Here's how to eyeball the perfect portion size every time. We give you two comparisons: One to everyday objects and the other to parts of your hand, for a take-anywhere system.

THE PERFECT PORTION	LOOKS LIKE THIS	OR THIS
3 ounces meat	A pack of tissues	Your outstretched palm
3 ounces fish	A checkbook	Your outstretched palm
1 cup beans	A tennis ball	A cupped handful
1½ ounces cheese	3 dice	Your thumb
2 tablespoons peanut butter	A golf ball	Your thumb
1 cup rice or pasta	A full cupcake wrapper	A rounded handful
1 small bagel	Diameter of a hockey puck	Your palm
1-ounce roll	A bar of soap	Half of your palm
1 small muffin	The round part of a lightbulb	Half of your fist
1 pancake or waffle	Diameter of a CD	Your palm with ½–1 inch overlap
3-by-3-inch piece of cake	A pack of Post-it notes	About ¾ of your palm
1 teaspoon butter or margarine	A postage stamp	The tip of your thumb
1 tablespoon oil or dressing	A silver dollar	The center of your cupped hand
Pretzels or chips	A tennis ball	A cupped handful
Nuts or dried fruit	A golf ball	A small cupped handful

Right-Size Your Meals

The good news: The volunteers were equally full and satisfied with any reasonable portion size—even when their entrées were prepared with fewer high-calorie ingredients. Here's how you can downsize your portions and still feel satisfied.

Contemplating seconds? Wait 10 minutes. Your stomach needs about that long to signal to the brain that it's full, so stall before helping yourself to more mashed potatoes or lasagna. Keep the conversation going, tell a joke, or, if you're dining alone, read the newspaper or walk around the house. If you're truly hungry after the delay, have seconds of the veggies or salad.

Quit the clean plate club. One in four Americans eat everything they're served no matter how big the portions, surveys reveal. A better strategy: Eat a healthy portion (see "Perfect Portion Size Guide" on page 94), then stop. It's better to waste a little food (or save it for tomorrow) than to overload your body.

***Never* eat directly out of the bag, box, or carton.** Put the right portion on a plate and put the package away, then sit down and enjoy.

Like big portions? Do this. Overload your plate with vegetables or salad with a smidgen of dressing or have a big, steaming bowl of broth-based soup, Dr. Rolls suggests. These water-rich, low-fat foods are so low in calories that a big portion isn't a problem.

Use a salad plate as your dinner plate. Less real estate means automatic portion control.

Make "small" your default setting. When ordering food or drinks or buying packaged food at the store, automatically go for the smallest size of any high-calorie items. (The exceptions: Salads and veggies without added fat.) Get the small latte, the 6-inch sub instead of the 12-inch, the small cookie instead of the 4-inch chocolate chip behemoth. Calories you haven't bought can't end up around your waist.

Go single-serve. Buy or make ice cream, sweets, or other high-cal foods, in individual serving sizes. Instead of a half-gallon of Rocky Road, buy ice cream sandwiches; make cupcakes instead of cake; and buy single-serving bags of chips.

But read the label first. Many packaged foods and drinks that look as if they provide one serving are actually meant to serve two or more people. However, the calories and other nutrition info on the label are for just one serving, so read the number of servings per container first. Then be sure to eat or drink just one serving.

Pack your leftovers before eating. Sure, it's easy to put a healthy plate of food in front of you. The trouble comes when the plate empties and you have more of each food sitting in front of you in alluring serving bowls. The answer: Package and store leftovers before you sit down to eat. That way, getting seconds becomes a whole lot harder and feels more inappropriate.

Round out the meal with raw produce. As you transition to more modest portion sizes, you may find yourself craving more food with your meal. The answer: a piece of fruit or a crunchy, large serving of celery, carrots, or peppers. There is no easier, healthier way to "beef up" a meal than with an apple, an orange, a big helping of watermelon or cantaloupe, or a sliced tomato.

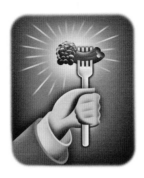

Superfoods to the Rescue

LUSCIOUS STRAWBERRIES dipped in rich, dark chocolate. Grilled salmon. Mashed sweet potatoes dusted with cinnamon. Spinach salad tossed with cranberries and walnuts. A gourmet's delight? Definitely. A huge dose of heart health—from good fats and fiber to powerful antioxidants and essential vitamins and minerals? Without a doubt.

Superfoods such as the 18 described below work better than supplements to slash your risk of heart disease. Not only do they entertain your taste buds like a four-star chef, they also battle all six deadly heart attackers at the same time. Specifically, the amazing foods in this chapter can:

- Reduce your risk of artery-clogging atherosclerosis
- Whittle away at cholesterol
- Lower your blood pressure
- Cool inflammation
- Neutralize damaging free radicals
- Reduce your chances of developing metabolic syndrome by keeping blood sugar lower and steadier
- When eaten in healthy portions, help you lose weight

You don't have to go to the health food store to find them; just wheel your cart through the supermarket. (Hint: Most are in the perimeter aisles, including the produce, meat, and dairy departments.) More good news: We've pulled together the quickest, tastiest ways to cook and serve these healing foods, from tried-and-true favorites to fresh, new ideas. Healthy eating doesn't have to take extra time out of your busy day—reaching for an ounce of dark chocolate or a fistful of walnuts is as quick as grabbing a bag of chips. And the taste? Out of this world.

1 ALMONDS

✓ **Super nutrients.** Monounsaturated fat, magnesium, calcium, potassium, fiber.

✓ **Serving size.** 1 ounce (about 24 almonds); 160 calories.

✓ **Benefits.** A single serving of these crunchy, protein-packed nuggets provides a whopping 9 grams of monounsaturated fat to help slash LDLs ("bad" cholesterol) and boost HDLs ("good" cholesterol). Simply choosing almonds instead of a doughnut, chips, or pretzels for two snacks a day could cut LDLs nearly by 10 percent. Almonds also pack 6 percent of your daily calcium quota and 20 percent of the magnesium you need—two minerals proven to help lower blood pressure. Bonus: You get 35 percent of the Daily Value (DV) for vitamin E, an artery-protecting antioxidant, as well as 3 grams of fiber. Just be sure to stop with one handful at snack time—advice that holds true for all nuts because they're calorie-dense.

GOOD IDEAS

• One serving of almonds fits neatly into an empty Altoids mints tin. Fill the tin each morning and slip it into your purse or briefcase.

• Toss some almonds into salads, stir-fries, fruit salad, or hot or cold cereal.

• Keep slivered and sliced almonds on hand (store them in the freezer for freshness) to add to vegetable dishes, muffins, and cookies.

2 APPLES

✓ **Super nutrients.** Antioxidants, fiber.

✓ **Serving size.** 1 medium; 80 calories.

✓ **Benefits.** Red Delicious, Granny Smith, and Gala apples earned spots on the USDA's top-20 list of antioxidant-rich foods thanks to hefty quantities of the flavonoid quercetin (flavonoids are natural chemicals in plants that, when in your bloodstream, remove free radical molecules, fight inflammation, and impede cancer). Bonus: Apples are a rich source of pectin, a soluble fiber. In a recent study at the University of California, Davis, people who ate two apples a day had fewer oxidized, artery-attacking LDLs than non-apple eaters.

GOOD IDEAS

• Chop an apple and add to hot cereal.

• For a portable snack, cut up an apple and place the slices in a zipper-lock plastic bag with 2 teaspoons of cinnamon. Carry it with you in an insulated lunch bag (with a freezer pack) to eat at lunch or as a snack. It tastes like apple pie, without the crust or the sugar.

• For a quick baked apple, core an apple, pack the center with raisins and walnuts, and dust with cinnamon. Place it in a bowl with 1/4 cup of orange juice, apple juice, or water and microwave on high for 5 minutes, or until done.

3 AVOCADOS

✓ **Super nutrients.** Omega-3 fatty acids, vitamin E, potassium.

✓ **Serving size.** ¼ to ½ fruit; about 150 calories.

✓ **Benefits.** In a study at Mexico's Instituto Mexicano del Seguro Social, women and men who ate one avocado a day for a week had reductions in total cholesterol of 17 percent. The amazing details: While their levels of unhealthy LDLs and triglycerides fell, beneficial HDLs actually rose—thanks, perhaps, to avocado's high levels of "good" monounsaturated fat. This fatty fruit is also full of a cholesterol-cutting nutrient called beta-sitosterol.

GOOD IDEAS

• Use mashed avocado in place of cheese, butter, or cream cheese. Although avocados provide good fat, there's 30 grams in a whole fruit (as much as in a quarter-pound hamburger), and they're loaded with calories. That's why it's a good idea to use it in place of another high-fat item instead of just adding half an avocado to your diet.

• Spread mashed avocado on bread.

• Mix it with lemon juice and chopped cilantro for homemade guacamole. Serve with baked chips.

• Chop and add to salads.

• Add slices to sandwiches.

• Stir cubes into chicken-rice soup.

4 BANANAS

✓ **Super nutrients.** Potassium, magnesium.

✓ **Serving size.** 1 medium; 105 calories.

✓ **Benefits.** Researchers from India found that people who ate two bananas a day cut their blood pressure levels by as much as 10 percent, thanks to this fruit's artery-relaxing potassium and magnesium. Potassium also helps regulate sodium and water content in the bloodstream—high levels of both raise blood pressure. (One caveat: If you have diabetes, check your blood sugar after eating a banana—its high carb count could send glucose soaring.)

GOOD IDEAS

• Spread banana slices with peanut butter for a luscious snack.

• Freeze a peeled banana for a treat that's 100 percent fruit.

• Use sliced banana in place of jelly on your next peanut butter sandwich.

• Add banana chunks to hot cereal while it is cooking.

All-American Superstar: The Peanut

A handful of roasted peanuts packs 62 milligrams of phytosterols—plant compounds that prevent your body from absorbing cholesterol and may help explain why women and men who regularly eat peanuts and other nuts have a 30 to 50 percent lower risk of fatal heart attacks. Peanuts are also a good source of homocysteine-lowering folate and blood pressure–regulating magnesium.

5 BERRIES, BERRIES, BERRIES!

✓ **Super nutrients.** Antioxidants, vitamin C, fiber.

✓ **Serving size.** ½ cup; about 60 calories

✓ **Benefits.** From wild blueberries and cranberries to strawberries, raspberries, and blackberries, these tiny but mighty fruits crowd the top of the USDA's latest list of antioxidant-rich foods. Inside each juicy bite: beneficial plant-based compounds such as quercetin, kaempferol, and anthocyanins (which give berries their brilliant red and blue hues) that act as antioxidants that can reduce the oxidation of LDLs and cool inflammation. Berries also contain salicylic acid, the same anti-inflammatory substance found in aspirin. Make every day berry-licious, regardless of the season

GOOD IDEAS

- Keep frozen berries in your freezer and add them to smoothies, hot cereal, and fruit salads.

- Make healthier soft-serve by whirling frozen berries, fat-free milk, and sugar substitute in the food processor.

- Add berries to tossed green salads or make an all-berry salad and dress it with lemon vinaigrette.

- Enjoy an elegant dessert: Simply top raspberries with 1 ounce of melted dark chocolate.

- Add berries to anything you cook with flour. Blueberries go great in breads made in bread machines, and raspberries add a unique twist to cookies. Also add berries to pancake, waffle, and muffin batters. Be sure to compensate for the moisture they add to the recipe by reducing the other liquids slightly.

Chocolate's a Health Food!

Just 1 ounce of luscious, dark chocolate packs as much as 41 milligrams of flavanols—powerful antioxidants that guard against plaque buildup in artery walls. That's a bigger antioxidant punch than a cup of green tea, an apple, or a goblet of red wine, and it's one that may also reduce blood clotting and help keep arteries flexible.

Before you rush to the all-night convenience store for any old chocolate bar, though, keep reading: To get chocolate's benefits, experts say to choose one with the highest cocoa content,

such as Dove Dark made with Cocoapro cocoa (it contains extra flavanols), Scharffen Berger Bittersweet, or El Rey Gran Saman Dark Chocolate. To get heart-healthy benefits without adding too much hip-padding fat, limit yourself to an ounce a day. Here are some ways to stretch your chocolate budget.

- Add citrus to unlock more of chocolate's antioxidant powers. In a saucepan, slowly heat a 14-ounce can of fat-free sweetened condensed milk with 6 ounces of semi-sweet chocolate chips. Peel eight tangerines, separate the sections, and dip them in the melted chocolate mixture. Serves eight.

- Spread 1 tablespoon of creamy or chunky peanut butter on 1 ounce of dark chocolate for a satisfying good-fat-packed treat.

- Start with pure cocoa powder (rather than a mix) when baking or making hot chocolate. It contains even more antioxidants than a chocolate bar.

6 BROCCOLI

✓ **Super nutrients.** Antioxidants, calcium, folate, glucoraphanin.

✓ **Serving size.** 1 medium stalk; 50 calories.

✓ **Benefits.** Glucoraphanin, a compound in broccoli shown to fight cancer, may also cut the risk of high blood pressure, cardiovascular disease, and stroke, studies suggest. Unlike antioxidant molecules that attack a single free radical and then lose their power, this powerful substance boosts the body's entire antioxidant defense system so that it can disarm *lots* of free radicals. Flavonoids in broccoli also cool inflammation and discourage formation of blood clots.

GOOD IDEAS

- Sprinkle finely chopped broccoli florets over casseroles, soups, and salads.

- Steam and refrigerate extra broccoli; tuck some into an omelet with a slice of low-fat cheese or serve it as a side dish at lunch.

- Skip high-fat, premade broccoli-and-cheese-sauce side dishes from the freezer case. Buy plain frozen broccoli, then heat it and top with grated Parmesan and a little olive oil.

- Add antioxidant-rich broccoli sprouts (available in the produce aisle) to salads and sandwiches.

- Puree cooked broccoli with olive oil, garlic, and crushed red pepper flakes to use as a sauce for pasta.

7 CARROTS

✓ **Super nutrients.** One of nature's top sources of beta-carotene, an artery-protecting antioxidant.

✓ **Serving size.** 1 medium; 32 calories.

✓ **Benefits.** Carrots are color therapy for your cardiovascular system. These veggies' brilliant orange hue is a sign of super-high levels of beta-carotene, an antioxidant that guards against artery-clogging oxidized LDL cholesterol. Only foods like carrots offer this protection—recent studies suggest that antioxidant pills don't help your heart. Cooked carrots have twice the antioxidant power of raw carrots because heat breaks down tough cell walls so that your body can use what's inside. Carrots also provide blood pressure–lowering potassium and magnesium, plus the homocysteine-lowering combination of folate; vitamin B_6; and the antioxidants alpha-carotene, lutein, and zeaxanthin.

GOOD IDEAS

- Set out a bowl of baby carrots when you're cooking as a healthy snack that won't fill you up with unwanted calories or wreck your appetite.

- Buy sliced and shredded carrots in the produce department; add them to soups, salads, and casseroles.

- Instead of chips, serve presliced carrots with dip.

- Add finely grated carrots to muffins, tuna or salmon salad, and casseroles.

- Microwave baby carrots and stir in a dollop of honey for a sweet side dish.

- Roast carrots in the oven with olive oil.

8 LEAN BEEF

✓ **Super nutrients.** Vitamin B_6, vitamin B_{12}, stearic acid.

✓ **Serving size.** 4 ounces; 240 calories.

✓ **Benefits.** In addition to its protein, a 4-ounce serving of lean beef provides nearly 122 percent of the DV for vitamin B_{12} and almost 38 percent of the DV for B_6. The body needs both these vitamins to convert homocysteine into other, benign molecules (high homocysteine levels are associated with increased risk of heart attack and stroke and with osteoporosis). And while beef is a major source of saturated fat, a third of it is stearic acid, which has a neutral or even beneficial effect on blood cholesterol levels.

GOOD IDEAS

- Look for the words "lean" or "extra-lean" on the label; these cuts have 4.5 grams or less of saturated fat and 5 to 10 grams of total fat per serving. Or look for these lean cuts: bottom, eye, or top round; round tip; top sirloin; and top loin or tenderloin.

- Sauté thin slices of steak with onions, garlic, and fresh basil and serve over brown rice.

- Add ground beef to tomato sauce and serve over pasta.

- Skewer beef cubes with your favorite vegetables, then brush with a little olive oil, and grill.

- Layer thinly sliced cooked tenderloin on toasted whole wheat French bread; top with roasted peppers and onions for a delicious open-faced sandwich.

- Coat steaks with crushed peppercorns before grilling.

The Cattle Controversy

In general, the beef on our dinner plates comes from cattle that are fed food you just don't want to know about and are kept in conditions you don't want to hear about. This is one reason that these days, the trendiest beef available in supermarkets (and from the Internet) comes from "free-ranging," grass-munching cows. Some grass-devoted cattlemen go a step further, offering meat from traditionally pastured "heirloom" cattle breeds such as Galloway, Hereford, Devon, and Highlander.

Is meat from grass-fed cattle worth the extra cost (prices range from about $4 a pound for a roast to $20 a pound for tenderloin)? That depends as much on your concern about animal treatment as it does on your concerns about health. Like plant-eating wild game, "pasture-raised" cattle may contain 50 to 85 percent more heart-healthy omega-3 fatty acids and less saturated fat than feedlot cattle raised on highly processed feed.

Some tasters say that grass-fed beef has a gamey or even bitter flavor, while enthusiasts say it tastes "beefier" than the roasts and steaks most of us grew up eating. What's more, the "grass-fed" description may be misleading. While some farmers do let their herds roam the pastures, others start their cattle on corn and processed feed and switch them to grass later. Your best bet: Before you buy pasture-raised beef, ask your supermarket's butcher about the producer. And have a pot roast recipe handy: Many cuts of grass-fed beef are extremely lean, and slow cooking tenderizes it.

9 MILK

✓ **Super nutrients.** Great source of blood pressure–lowering calcium, magnesium, and potassium.

✓ **Serving size.** 8 ounces 1% milk; 110 calories.

✓ **Benefits.** Your heart—and your waist-line—love it when you have a milk mustache. (So, of course, do your bones!) A growing stack of research proves that calcium and other minerals in milk help lower blood pressure by keeping arteries flexible and helping your kidneys flush pressure-boosting sodium out of your body. A glass of cold moo juice at lunch or a generous splash on your morning cereal could cut your risk of insulin resistance—a potent heart disease risk factor— by 71 percent *and* help you lose weight. How? Mayo Clinic researchers suspect that calcium "down-regulates" fat absorption by fat cells and "up-regulates" fat burning.

GOOD IDEAS

- A favorite cocoa recipe: Mix 1 cup of fat-free or low-fat milk, two packets of sugar substitute, and cocoa in a small saucepan or microwaveable cup and heat for about 1 minute.

- Cook hot cereal and low-sodium instant or canned soups with milk instead of water.

- Make milk your drive-through thirst quencher. Most fast-food restaurants offer the low-fat variety in cartons or single-serve bottles.

- Order a latte with fat-free milk instead of black or with cream at your favorite coffee shop.

Hydrate Your Heart

Sparkling or still, bottled or straight from the tap, water is kind to your heart: Sipping at least five glasses a day could cut your risk of a deadly heart attack by as much as 54 percent, report researchers from Loma Linda University in California. In their study of 20,000 women and men, they found that those who wet their whistles with other beverages—from coffee to OJ—had higher heart attack risks.

H_2O's superpower? It's absorbed readily into the bloodstream, so it keeps blood diluted and less likely to form heart-threatening clots. Other liquids, the researchers say, require digestion, a process that draws fluid out of the bloodstream, thus thickening the blood and increasing the risk of clots.

- Make sugar-free instant pudding with low-fat or fat-free milk and serve it with berries.

- Use fat-free evaporated milk in place of regular milk in baked goods, soups, and sauces. A cup contains 742 milligrams of calcium—more than double the amount in low-fat milk.

- Whip partially frozen fat-free evaporated milk for a high-calcium dessert topping that has one-tenth the calories of regular whipped cream.

- Puree fat-free or low-fat cottage cheese and fat-free evaporated milk with some lemon juice and rosemary for a light pasta sauce.

10 KIDNEY BEANS

✓ **Super nutrients.** Soluble fiber, folate, potassium, magnesium.

✓ **Serving size.** ½ cup; 112 calories.

✓ **Benefits.** Eating beans four times a week—in baked beans, bean dip, chili, or a salad sprinkled with chickpeas or black beans—could cut your risk of coronary heart disease by 20 to 30 percent. Make some of them kidney beans; they're rich in LDL-lowering soluble fiber (2 grams in a 1/2-cup serving) and homocysteine-controlling folate, as well as blood pressure–easing potassium and magnesium. Bonus: Thanks to healthy doses of fiber and protein, beans give you steady energy, not a sudden rise (and fall) of blood sugar that ups your risk of metabolic syndrome and weight gain.

GOOD IDEAS

• Rinse canned kidney beans before using to remove sodium. Toss them into chili, casseroles, and soups.

• For a quick tamale pie, serve warm kidney beans over a piece of cornbread and top with grated cheese.

• Make a better three-bean salad: Combine kidney, black, and white beans, then mix in chopped tomatoes and scallions. Dress with olive oil, lemon juice, and black pepper.

• In a food processor or blender, combine cooked kidney beans with garlic, cumin, and chili peppers for a delicious spread that can be used as a dip for crudités or a sandwich filling.

11 WALNUTS

✓ **Super nutrients.** More omega-3 fatty acids than any other nut.

✓ **Serving size.** 1 ounce (14 halves); 190 calories.

✓ **Benefits.** One serving of walnuts contains 2.6 grams of alpha-linolenic acid (ALA), an omega-3 fatty acid that helps prevent blood clots and promote a healthy heartbeat. Walnuts are also rich in vitamin B_6, which helps control homocysteine. In one study, people who consumed 1.6 ounces of walnuts every day for six weeks cut levels of extra-harmful very low density lipoproteins by 27 percent. These delicious nuts also provide the amino acid arginine, which helps your body produce nitric acid, a molecule that relaxes constricted blood vessels.

GOOD IDEAS

• Chop walnuts in a food processor with a dollop of canola oil and a generous helping of cinnamon. Spread over chopped fruit in a baking dish and bake for 45 minutes at 350°F for a healthy fruit crisp.

• Keep a jar of chopped walnuts in the freezer to toss into cold or hot cereal, baked goods, pancakes, and waffles.

• Treat yourself to a nut snack at mid-morning or midafternoon: Drop 14 walnut halves into a zipper-lock bag and carry it with you.

12 OATMEAL

✓ **Super nutrients.** Cholesterol-lowering soluble fiber, plus slow-release carbs that won't make your blood sugar spike.

✓ **Serving size.** 1 to 1½ cups cooked; 145 to 210 calories.

✓ **Benefits.** Beta-glucan, the soluble fiber in oats, acts like a sponge in your intestines, absorbing cholesterol-rich bile acids and eliminating them. The result is lower LDLs. Having a big bowl of oatmeal (1½ cups) each day could cut cholesterol by 2 to 3 percent, suggests a study published in the *Journal of the American Medical Association*. Soluble fiber may also lower blood pressure.

GOOD IDEAS

- Flavor it yourself: Buy old-fashioned, quick-cooking, or plain (no sugar added) instant oatmeal instead of flavored instant oatmeal. Add brown sugar or maple syrup, dried or fresh fruit, nuts, and milk.

- For flaky (versus creamy) oatmeal, bring a saucepan of water to a boil, add old-fashioned oats, and bring back to a rolling boil. Turn off the heat, and cover the pan. In 10 minutes, the oatmeal will be ready to eat.

- Replace up to one-third of the flour in pancake recipes with oatmeal; grind it into a fine powder first in the blender.

- Use oatmeal to thicken soups and stews by just tossing in a handful.

- For a heart-healthy streusel topping for fruit, combine chopped walnuts, a dollop of canola oil, oats, and brown sugar to taste. Spread over cut fruit in a baking dish and bake at 350°F for 30 to 45 minutes.

9 Surprising Uses for Cinnamon

A half-teaspoon of cinnamon each day—sprinkled on your morning toast or spicing up steamed carrots—could cut your triglycerides and total cholesterol by 12 to 30 percent, report researchers at the USDA Beltsville Human Nutrition Research Center in Maryland.

This pungent spice makes muscle and liver cells more sensitive to the hormone insulin, reducing the insulin resistance that can throw blood fats (and blood sugar) out of whack. Here are ways to sneak more of this amazingly heart-healthy spice into your diet.

1. Sprinkle a little in your morning coffee or cocoa.
2. Double the amount called for in muffin, pie, and cookie recipes.
3. Use in place of salt and pepper on baked sweet potatoes.
4. Create zero-carb cinnamon-sugar: Make a 2-to-1 mixture of cinnamon and a sugar substitute such as Splenda to use on oatmeal, toast, and even scrambled eggs.
5. Add it to chili and curries for an authentic flavor.
6. Create sweet breakfast rice by stirring raisins, nuts, and cinnamon into reheated leftover brown rice.
7. Stir it into marinades for beef, pork, or lamb.
8. Stuff a chicken or Cornish hen with chopped apples, cinnamon, onion, and a little sage.
9. In a small baking dish, toss 2 cups of pecans with 3 teaspoons of canola oil, 2 teaspoons of cinnamon, and 1 teaspoon of sugar substitute or sugar. Bake at 350°F for 8 to 10 minutes.

13 SALMON

✓ **Super nutrients.** Richest source of omega-3 fatty acids.

✓ **Serving size.** 3 to 4 ounces (about the size of your palm); about 230 calories.

✓ **Benefits.** Among omega-3–rich fatty fish, salmon is king: One serving contains nearly 2 grams of eicosapentaenoic acid (EPA) and docosahexaenoic acid (DHA), important omega-3s that help cut your risk of deadly, out-of-rhythm heartbeats; reduce LDLs (especially extra-dangerous very low density lipoproteins that clog arteries easily); cool inflammation; and may even discourage atherosclerosis and the formation of heart-threatening blood clots.

The American Heart Association recommends that everyone eat fish at least twice a week; other experts suggest that having four servings per week is even healthier.

GOOD IDEAS

- Check on the source of the salmon. In 2003, lab tests conducted by the non-profit Environmental Working Group found that farm-raised salmon (as opposed to ocean-caught salmon) may have levels of contaminants called poly-chlorinated biphenyls (PCBs) that are 7 to 16 times higher than those in wild salmon. This could change quickly now that the problem has been identified and salmon farmers are addressing the issue, so monitor the news for the newest test results.

- Go for canned salmon. While wild salmon fillets and steaks are difficult to find in most supermarkets (and may cost as much as $28 per pound), canned salmon is a brilliant alternative. It is wild

The Truth About Mercury

Most fish contains trace amounts of mercury, which pose little danger to adults but can stunt brain and nervous system growth in babies and young children. Hence the FDA's fish-intake recommendations for pregnant and nursing moms, women trying to become pregnant, and kids under age 5.

- Limit low-mercury seafood such as shrimp, salmon, pollock, and "light" tuna to two meals per week.

- Eat higher-mercury albacore tuna (the can may say "solid" or "chunk" white) no more than once a week. Organizations such as the Environmental Working Group advise pregnant women to avoid all canned tuna.

- Don't eat shark, swordfish, king mackerel, or tilefish, which all contain high levels of mercury.

salmon, yet it usually costs less than $5 per can. Use it in place of tuna to make salmon salad, toss it with pasta, add it to casseroles, or try our recipe for salmon patties on page 249.

- Order wild salmon when dining out. With more eateries offering this treat, don't pass it up when you're having a special dinner out. It's a great way to fit in an extra fish serving.

Soy for Beginners

Soy foods—from milk to soy nuts—may help lower heart-damaging LDLs, thanks to unique plant estrogens called genistein and daidzen. Soy has become so mainstream that the American Heart Association recommends it as part of a heart-healthy diet, and the FDA allows some soy products to carry a special "heart healthy" claim on their labels.

Yet not everyone's sold on soy. While some experts recommend two to four servings a week, one recent study found that soy offered no heart protection for postmenopausal women. (Skip soy entirely if you're taking a breast cancer prevention drug, such as tamoxifen, or medication for low thyroid.) Still, it may be helpful for some people. If you're new to soy, here are six ways to give it a whirl.

Edamame. That's the Japanese name for fresh soybeans. They resemble peas in shape, size, and color and come in pods just like sweet peas. Usually, you buy them frozen in the vegetable section of well-stocked supermarkets; they're available in the pod or already shelled. Steam them and eat the beans unadorned or with a pinch of salt. Not only are they absolutely delicious, but in this form, soy most closely resembles regular American vegetables.

Miso soup. This delicate and delectable soup made from soybeans is often the first course of a Japanese-style dinner. Today, supermarkets carry miso soup packets that are as cheap and easy as any "noodles in a cup" product. Just pour the contents of the packet into a cup of hot water, stir, and voilà—you have a wonderful, quick soup. Have some instead of coffee or as a warm-me-up on cold days.

Calcium-fortified soy milk. High in protein, calcium, and isoflavones (plant chemicals that act like the hormone estrogen in the body), fortified soy milk can substitute for cow's milk in coffee or tea or on breakfast cereal.

Soy nuts. Dry-roasted soy nuts are among the richest sources of soy isoflavones. Grab a handful as an afternoon snack or toss some into a salad. You'll find them in health food stores.

Soy burgers and hot dogs. Look for the FDA-approved heart-health claim on the label, a sign that the product contains at least 6.25 grams of soy protein per serving. (Skip items that don't have the heart-health label. Some soy cold cuts, burgers, pocket sandwiches, and frozen entrées may be high in fat, loaded with trans fats, and/or contain few isoflavones.)

Textured vegetable protein (TVP). Okay, TVP does sound a bit odd: It's defatted, dehydrated soy flour that's been compressed into tiny clumps and chunks. If you soak it (stir 1 cup of TVP into $7/8$ cup of hot water or broth and drain after 5 to 10 minutes) and add it to chili, sloppy Joes or tacos, it has the chewy texture of ground meat. Bonus: Lots of isoflavones. Uncooked TVP will keep in a cool, dark pantry for months.

14 SPINACH

✓ **Super nutrients.** Folate, magnesium, potassium.

✓ **Serving size.** 1 cup raw, 6 calories; ½ cup cooked, 40 calories.

✓ **Benefits.** Spinach is brimming with 58 micrograms of folate per cup of raw leaves. Getting 300 milligrams per day of this essential nutrient could cut your heart disease risk by 13 percent. A half-cup of cooked spinach provides 502 milligrams of blood pressure–controlling potassium, too.

GOOD IDEAS

- No time to painstakingly rinse and trim each leaf in a bagful of fresh spinach? Grabbing a microwaveable bag of pre-washed stuff is worth the added expense. Slit the bag, add a dollop of olive oil and some chopped garlic, then follow the heat-and-eat directions.

- Want a spinach salad? Rinse some pre-washed spinach to clean away germs, then toss it with walnuts, cranberries, and sliced precooked chicken for a fast, healthy dinner.

- Add spinach to homemade soup or jazz up canned soup. Stir it in just before you turn off the heat.

- Layer spinach on sandwiches instead of lettuce.

15 TURKEY

✓ **Super nutrients.** Protein, vitamin B$_6$, vitamin B$_{12}$, niacin.

✓ **Serving size.** 4 ounces; 214 calories

✓ **Benefits.** Don't save roast turkey for your Thanksgiving feast. A 4-ounce serving provides more than 60 percent of the hunger-satisfying, blood sugar–controlling protein you need in one day, with only half the saturated fat found in most cuts of red meat. And it's packed with homocysteine-lowering niacin, plus vitamins B$_6$ and B$_{12}$. This trio helps your body convert carbs, fats, and protein into energy. Luckily, you don't have to buy a 22-pound turkey to reap these benefits, since turkey is becoming increasingly available cut up into reasonably sized portions or as ground meat.

GOOD IDEAS

- Use skinless ground turkey instead of ground beef or ground chicken in recipes for chili, meat loaf, and burgers.

- Grill or bake a turkey breast instead of a whole chicken. Slice, then refrigerate or freeze leftovers to use in turkey burritos or turkey salad (toss diced turkey with low-fat mayo, chopped apples, walnuts, celery, and grapes).

- Make Thanksgiving salad: Place some cubed turkey, sliced cooked sweet potato, cranberries, and walnuts on a bed of spinach and drizzle with your favorite olive oil dressing.

- Keep skinless, boneless turkey cutlets in the freezer for quick meals. Thaw them in the microwave, then sauté with a dollop of olive oil and your favorite seasonings.

16 TOMATOES

✓ **Super nutrients.** Lycopene, fiber, vitamin C.

✓ **Serving size.** 1 cup sliced tomatoes, ½ cup sauce, or ¾ cup low-sodium tomato juice; 40 to 60 calories.

✓ **Benefits.** Fresh from the vine, cooked down into a thick sauce, or sun dried, tomatoes are the wonder veggie. Eating seven or more servings per week cut risk of cardiovascular disease 30 percent in a recent study of more than 35,000 women conducted by doctors at Boston's Brigham and Women's Hospital. The heart-smart factor? It could be the antioxidant lycopene or tomatoes' stellar levels of vitamin C, potassium, and fiber. An interesting note: Tomatoes that have been cooked for 30 minutes (as they are for sauce, puree, paste, and salsa) have significantly higher levels of lycopene than raw tomatoes. And 1/4 cup of sun-dried tomatoes has more potassium than a medium banana.

GOOD IDEAS

- For tasty, fresh tomatoes when tomato season's past, try grape, plum, or on-the-vine types from the produce department. Give 'em the sniff test: If they smell like ripe tomatoes, chances are they'll taste good, too.

- Toss a handful of sun-dried tomatoes into chili or casseroles or while sautéing chicken or salmon. They're also delicious cooked with chopped garlic, a little olive oil, and a splash of white wine.

Organic—Or Not?

If the promise of food untainted by chemical pesticides and fertilizers isn't enough incentive to choose organically grown foods, consider this: Scottish and American studies suggest that organic fruits and veggies may be richer in calcium; iron; phosphorus; zinc; and vitamins A, C, and E than conventionally grown produce. The rest of the story is that going organic could double or triple your produce bill—but you can shop healthy without blowing the grocery budget. Choose organic versions of produce known to carry higher levels of pesticide residue and stick with conventionally grown varieties for the rest. Here's how to choose.

Produce with often-high levels of pesticide residue
Apples, bell peppers, celery, cherries, imported grapes, nectarines, peaches, pears, raspberries, strawberries, tomatoes

Produce with low levels of pesticide residue
Asparagus, avocados, bananas, blueberries, broccoli, cabbage, cauliflower, eggplant, grapefruit, kiwifruit, mangoes, onions, plums, radishes, watermelon

- For quick chili, combine the following ingredients in a glass bowl and heat in the microwave: canned, rinsed black beans; tomato sauce; frozen corn; and a dash of cumin and oregano.

- Blessed with a bountiful harvest from your vegetable garden? Core big tomatoes, add a scoop of tuna or salmon salad, and serve.

17 SWEET POTATOES

✓ **Super nutrients.** Beta-carotene, fiber, antioxidants.

✓ **Serving size.** One medium; 117 calories.

✓ **Benefits.** Rated the number-one health-iest vegetable by Nutrition Action Health Letter, a sweet potato is nearly a meal in itself —full of protein, fiber, artery-pro-tecting beta-carotene, blood pressure–controlling potassium, and antioxi-dant vitamins C and E. Unlike white potatoes, sweet potatoes won't send your blood sugar soaring.

GOOD IDEAS

- Wash and pierce the skin of two sweet potatoes and microwave on high for 6 to 8 minutes. Mash with a dollop of olive oil for a savory tater or with cinnamon and a teaspoon of brown sugar for a very sweet treat.

- Toss a peeled, cubed sweet potato with a little olive oil in a small baking dish. Roast at 450°F, stirring frequently until slightly browned.

- Whip up a healthy, tastier alternative to regular fries: Slice four sweet potatoes, toss with 3 tablespoons of canola oil, spread on baking sheets, and bake at 425°F until tender, about 20 minutes. For sweet fries, sprinkle with cinnamon. For savory fries, sprinkle with a mixture of 1 teaspoon each of cumin and salt plus ½ teaspoon ground red pepper.

The Art and Science of Tea

Every day, it seems, science reconfirms that tea—whether it's a trendy green brew or traditional black tea—is a heart helper. A huge, 12-year Japanese study found that men who drank at least 32 ounces of green tea each day cut their risk of dying from cardiovascular disease by 42 percent. Antioxidants called catechins in green tea play a role in reducing the negative effects of bad cholesterol, lowering triglyceride levels, and increasing the production of good cholesterol.

Drinking three cups of black tea a day could lower heart attack risk by 30 percent, Dutch researchers discovered. Lab studies suggest that theaflavins—antioxidants found even in regular supermarket tea brands—can cut levels of "bad" LDL choles-terol by 16 to 24 percent. Black tea also makes arteries more flexible.

Which should you drink? Let your taste buds decide. Here's what you need to know.

Green tea. Delicately flavored, green tea is less processed, less caffeinated, more subtle, and less colorful than black tea. If you're new to green tea, try a variety flavored with fruit, honey, or spices. Note: Even ready-made green tea drinks (buy a sugar-free variety) are heart healthy.

Black tea. You don't have to special-order it from China; supermarket varieties are perfectly fine. For variety, experiment with naturally flavored types such as flowery Earl Grey or citrusy, spicy Russian Caravan. For iced tea tomorrow, add six tea bags to a quart of cool water, cover, and refrigerate overnight.

18 WATERMELON

✓ **Super nutrients.** Lycopene, potassium.

✓ **Serving size.** 1- by 10-inch slice; about 84 calories.

✓ **Benefits.** Don't save this gorgeous melon for summer; the salad bar in your supermarket probably has watermelon for much of the year. One slice packs more blood pressure–lowering potassium than an average banana (559 milligrams vs. 451 milligrams). Also inside: lots of antioxidant lycopene. Harvard researchers reported that women with the most lycopene in their blood had a 50 percent lower risk of heart disease than those who had the least.

- Add cubes or balls of watermelon to fruit salad. (Buy a melon-ball cutter in the supermarket; scooping out balls is quicker than cutting up a melon.)

- Freeze chunks of watermelon, then whirl in a food processor with sugar substitute for fresh watermelon ice.

- Make melon kabobs by alternating cubes of watermelon, cooked low-sodium turkey breast, and low-fat cheese on wooden skewers.

- Add watermelon chunks to chicken salad or green salads.

5 Heart-Healthy Switches

Make these easy food switches, and you'll automatically cut your risk of heart disease significantly. **1.** Cook and bake with olive and canola oils. Toss out the other vegetable oils in your cupboard; unlike canola oil, which is rich in omega-3 fatty acids, they contain high levels of omega-6 fatty acids that can promote inflammation. And they don't offer as much monounsaturated fat, which protects "good" HDL cholesterol, as olive oil. When baking, experiment with the least amount of butter or tub margarine you can use. Try replacing half with canola oil.

2. Go for brown starches. Buy brown rice, whole grain hot cereal, and whole wheat pasta (or a whole wheat/refined wheat mix) instead of the white varieties. You'll get heart-healthy fiber and antioxidants, such as natural vitamin E, and you will help control blood sugar spikes that lead to hunger and ultimately raise the risk of heart disease and diabetes.
3. Prepare hot cereals and soups (when appropriate) with low-fat or fat-free milk instead of water. You'll get an extra serving of blood pressure–lowering calcium.

4. Always add extra veggies to soups, stews, and casseroles. When heating canned soups, stir in some frozen veggies. If you're making homemade soup or stew, prepare twice the amount of vegetables called for. Cook and puree half and add them to the dish, then cook the rest as directed.
5. Keep a covered container of washed, bite-size fruit (cut fruit or grapes or berries) in the fridge. Put it on the counter while you're making a meal and on the table when you serve it. Just by nibbling, you'll get an extra fruit serving per day.

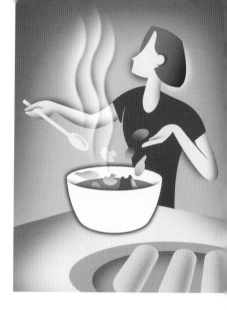

Cooking Cures

HOMEMADE *IS* HEALTHIER. We eat 50 percent less calories, fat, and sodium when we eat at home than when we eat out, notes the American Dietetic Association, the nation's premier source of nutritional knowledge. And that's not all: Gathering around the kitchen table virtually guarantees that you and your family will eat more fruits, veggies, whole grains, beans, and other nutrient-packed, heart-healthy power foods than you would at a burger chain or even a sit-down restaurant.

Nevertheless, lots of obstacles can get in the way of putting a healthy breakfast, lunch, or dinner on the table. Among them: A busy schedule; high-calorie cooking habits; a family who wants the old meals back (or would rather eat out); and reliance on processed, premade convenience foods. Discouraged? Don't be. We've got the solutions.

These cooking cures won't take any more time (and may actually take less) than you're spending now to make a meal. What's more, most may save you money because they rely on healthy, quick-cooking, minimally processed foods instead of expensive processed entrées and side dishes.

Use lots of precut, prewashed, and/or frozen fruits and veggies

The cure for: Thrown-together dinners that feature no produce because you don't have the time or energy to buy, clean, chop, and cook it.

Heart-healthy bonus: Frozen veggies and fruits have as many, and sometimes more, nutrients than fresh because they're usually frozen soon after picking, when nutrient content is highest. Precut produce is also usually as nutritious as fresh.

The plan: Load your refrigerator with precut, prewashed, and/or frozen veggies, as well as frozen berries (and in winter, other frozen fruits, such as peaches). These convenient veggies cook up fast in the microwave, and having a variety on hand could double or triple a meal's veggie servings because it's so easy to open the bag, heat, and eat. Smart choices include baby carrots (easy to munch raw or cook in the microwave); sliced carrots, precut broccoli and cauliflower; and frozen blends of diced onions, garlic, and peppers.

Frozen berries don't even need to be defrosted; just let them thaw while you eat dinner, or mix the contents with other, room-temperature fruits.

Invest in a Slow Cooker

Opening the kitchen door on a cold day and sniffing the aroma of homemade chicken soup or beef stew is one of life's simple pleasures—and it's one you can enjoy even if you can't afford a full-time cook to rustle up meals for you. Instead, try a slow cooker. Powered by less electricity than it would take to cook the same meal in an electric oven, a slow cooker can turn a handful of ingredients into a one-pot feast while you're out working, shopping, visiting, or playing.

The most successful slow-cooker recipes are for dishes that have high moisture content, such a stews, chili, and roasted meat with veggies and sauce. (A slow cooker's low heat, generally between 170°F and 280°F, tenderizes lean cuts of beef or chicken.)

Here's the easiest way to cook a basic meal: Use bite-size chunks of meat (thaw them if they're frozen). If you have time, brown the meat the night before, then refrigerate. In the morning, add vegetables to the cooker first (they cook more slowly than meat and need to be closer to the heat source), then add the meat and some low-sodium chicken stock, garlic, fresh herbs, and a little white or red wine. Cover and cook on low for 8 hours, or on high for 5. Before serving, stir a little Dijon mustard into the sauce.

Stock your pantry for heart-healthy "magic meals"

The cure for: Nights when you're too tired to even figure out what's for dinner, and you've prepared nothing in advance.

Heart-healthy bonus: Fiber to lower cholesterol, spices and flavorings rich in antioxidants, good fats to please the palate and protect against atherosclerosis, and calcium to help control blood pressure.

The plan: Think like a short-order gourmet cook, and you could sit down to a cheese omelet with a spinach, mandarin orange, and pecan salad on the side; pasta with clam sauce and mushrooms and a glass of merlot; bean burritos with guacamole; and more—in just 15 minutes. The key? Your imagination—and a pantry stocked with healthy basics and a few fun, high-flavor extras.

By keeping quick-cooking items (such as eggs high in omega-3 fatty acids; whole wheat pastas; nuts; canned beans; canned seafood; whole grain breads; and reduced-fat, low-sodium cheese) on hand, you'll be ready to whip up something fast and flavorful even on nights when you're drop-dead tired—the nights when you most need a good meal and are most vulnerable to eating too much of the wrong stuff. Here are four more fast, flavorful ideas.

- **Supercharged soup.** Add rinsed, canned beans and frozen veggies to low-sodium canned minestrone or vegetable soup. Serve with whole grain toast and a fruit salad (canned fruit mixed with frozen berries).

- **Field greens with chicken.** Rinse bagged spinach, arrange it on a plate, and top with nuts, precut carrots, and cherry tomatoes. Add strips of pre-cooked chicken breast and dress with olive oil and balsamic vinegar. Have sliced melon for dessert.

- **Simple pasta with white beans.** Cook whole wheat spaghetti, then toss with olive oil; Parmesan cheese; black pepper; and rinsed, heated canned white beans. Serve with steamed broccoli and fruit. (Variation: Toss the spaghetti and beans with a spoonful of pesto from a jar.)

- **Turkey melt with cranberry sauce on whole wheat.** Arrange sliced turkey on whole wheat bread and top with cranberry sauce and one slice of reduced-fat, low-sodium cheese. Microwave until the cheese melts. Serve with a green salad

Magic Pantry/Fridge Makeover

With the following items on hand, you can prepare healthy dinners in a flash.

- Brown rice
- Canned beans (black, navy, pinto, and kidney beans; chickpeas)
- Canned fruit in its own juice
- Canned salmon (red salmon is tastiest)
- Canned tomatoes
- Canola oil
- Dried fruit (especially raisins)
- Garlic (fresh and/or a jar of minced)
- Low-sodium chicken, beef, or vegetable broth
- Olive oil
- Onions
- Pasta sauce (7 percent saturated fat per serving)
- Peanut butter
- Salad dressings (made with canola or olive oil)
- Whole grain pasta
- Whole grain cereals (including oatmeal)

- Condiments (whatever you like, such as horseradish, salsa, mustards, ketchup, canola oil mayonnaise, fat-free sour cream, cranberry sauce, pesto in a jar, olives, capers, roasted red peppers packed in water, artichokes packed in water, chutney, jars of chopped garlic and ginger)
- Eggs (look for brands with extra-high levels of omega-3 fatty acids)
- Lots of fresh fruit
- Lots of fresh vegetables (including precut, prewashed produce)
- Low-fat or fat-free milk
- Low-fat or fat-free yogurt (plain and flavored)
- Parmesan cheese
- Reduced-fat, low-sodium cheeses

- Fish
- Frozen fruits (especially berries)
- Frozen vegetables
- Lean meats and poultry

and top off the meal with mixed berries and a dollop of low-fat frozen yogurt.

Make small changes

The cure for: A pretty good diet that could use a nutritional upgrade—more fruit and veggies, more fiber, more good fats, more dairy, or whatever applies to you.

Heart-healthy bonus: These changes are small enough, and tasty enough, that you'll soon make them part of your cooking repertoire—giving your cardiovascular system a steady dose of antioxidants, good fats, and vitamins and minerals.

The plan: You don't have to overhaul your kitchen and cooking style to eat for a healthy heart. Start with these smart cooking cures.

- Garnish fruit salads, green salads, and cooked veggies with chopped nuts for an extra helping of monounsaturated fats. Toss a handful into muffin and pancake recipes or add some to yogurt. For extra flavor, first toast the nuts in a 350°F oven until golden, 5 to 10 minutes.

- Top salads with avocado slices, rich in monounsaturated fat. Skip the bacon bits and croutons, which are dripping with saturated fat and trans fats.

- Instead of ice cream topped with a few strawberries, have a bowl of berries crowned with ½ cup of low-fat ice cream, frozen yogurt, or sorbet. You'll triple the antioxidants and cut your fat and sugar intake in half.

- Cook or serve veggies with a drizzle of olive or canola oil. Fat helps your body absorb more of the antioxidants, vitamins, and minerals in vegetables.

- Think in color. Serve fruits or veggies in contrasting colors: red peppers with broccoli, blueberries with peaches, or carrots and peas. New research suggests that the antioxidants in vegetables and fruits work harder when they're combined.

- Use canned salmon instead of tuna in your lunchtime "tuna salad" for a hefty dose of omega-3 fatty acids.

- Toss rinsed, canned beans into everyday foods—chickpeas on salad and kidney beans in spaghetti sauce. Beans are rich in appetite-controlling fiber.

- Keep a jar of minced garlic and a jar of minced ginger in the fridge. Use each at least once a week to season veggies, meats, or soups. Garlic may help lower cholesterol and cut the rate of plaque buildup in arteries, and antioxidant-rich ginger fights inflammation and may discourage formation of blood clots.

- Pump up your iron intake by cooking regularly in a cast-iron skillet or Dutch oven. Long-simmering soups, stews, and sauces absorb the most iron, but even scrambling an egg in a cast-iron skillet doubles the egg's iron content. Your body needs adequate iron to deliver oxygen to cells, including heart muscle cells.

- In recipes, cut the amount of salt in half or eliminate it entirely. Replace it with antioxidant-rich spices, garlic, or salt-free seasoning mixes.

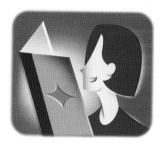

Managing Restaurants

AMERICA'S 800,000 restaurants are beckoning—from down-home diners and fast-food burger joints to Asian buffets and the hushed-and-haughty eateries of celebrity chefs. These days, most of us spend half the family grocery budget on food cooked behind closed doors in restaurant kitchens—but we're getting more than convenience and pleasure. Eating out—or bringing home takeout meals—doubles your intake of waistline-threatening calories, artery-clogging saturated fat and trans fats, and blood pressure–raising sodium.

The answer? If you expect us to suggest that you boycott local restaurants or adopt a dour "dry toast and steamed broccoli, please" attitude, you're in for a surprise.

On the 30-Minutes-A-Day Plan, you can eat restaurant food and takeout when you need to *and* when you want to—and

have a healthy, enjoyable experience. You won't have to call ahead to quiz the cook about calorie counts, limit yourself to the dieter's special, or pack your own salad dressing and sugar substitute. Why? We've discovered that by employing a few tricks, you can relax and savor a special dinner out, a business lunch, or Friday night pizza. You'll not only outsmart the heart attackers, you'll actually *nourish* your cardiovascular system. Here's how.

Before You Leave Home

Putting yourself in a healthy and fun mindset before you sit down (or pick up the phone) guarantees success. You'll avoid the pitfalls of restaurant food without feeling deprived. How? By refocusing on the great stuff you *can* have. Here's the strategy.

Imagine your meal. Picture your plate before you pick up the phone to order takeout, before you make a dinner reservation, and before getting out of your car at the diner on Saturday morning. Think creatively about the healthy options hiding out on most menus—the thin-crust pizza loaded with veggies, the fancy mixed-greens-and-pecans salad with vinaigrette on the side at the café downtown, or the incredible broiled fish at your local seafood restaurant.

Have fun treating yourself to good-for-you choices you might not cook at home, from roasted beets to wild salmon to exotic and wonderfully crunchy Chinese veggies, such as snow peas, bok choy, baby corn, and water chestnuts. And, if you absolutely must have a sweet treat once in a while, plan on splitting one when you go out to eat—your sweet tooth will be satisfied, and you won't have to deal with the temptation of leftover desserts in your own kitchen.

Don't skimp on breakfast and lunch. "Banking" extra calories before a big night out sounds smart, but this plan's got a tragic flaw: You're ravenous and ready to overeat by the time you arrive at the restaurant (or open the pizza box at the kitchen table). A better plan: *Spoil* your appetite by having nice daytime meals and then a hard-boiled egg and a piece of fruit, some yogurt and whole wheat toast, or a bowl of whole grain cereal with low-fat milk before heading to the restaurant. Worried about the extra calories and fat? Consider this: A smart snack at home is bound to have fewer calories and more nutrients than most restaurant appetizers.

Extra credit: Walk to the restaurant. If you can safely stroll from your home

Transform Your Takeout

Cut the calories and the fat, without cutting the flavor.

Pizza: Ask for thin crust, half the cheese, double the tomato sauce, and order lots of veggie toppings.

Chinese: Pick one chicken or shrimp dish for every two or three people, plus one order of steamed veggies. At home, put the veggies in a big bowl and spoon the entrée items on top, leaving the sauce—a big source of fat—behind in the original container. If your crowd loves rice, be sure to order brown rice.

Sandwiches: Eat 'em open-faced to save 80 to 90 calories. Skip the mayo and go with mustard as your first choice, ketchup as your second, or olive oil and herbs as your third. Ask for extra tomatoes, lettuce, and onions. Lean toward turkey, chicken, or roast beef, since processed meats such as salami are extremely high in fat, and tuna salad is often pure mayonnaise when made at a restaurant.

Mexican: No hard taco shells or tortilla chips; instead, choose soft tacos and burritos. Hold the sour cream and guacamole, but add lots and lots of salsa. If you have a choice, take black beans over refried beans.

to your destination, do so. Other options: Arrive early, then take a walk with your dinner companions, or go for a short jaunt after you eat. You'll burn extra calories and place the emphasis where it belongs: on socializing, not just on food.

At the Restaurant

When ordering, don't feel shy about asking questions and making special requests to ensure that your meal is exactly what you want. Your server is the link between table and kitchen. Make her—or him—your ally. Of course, don't be shy about tipping a helpful server, either.

These tricks will help you avoid empty calories, leaving you free to enjoy your meal without guilt.

Banish the bread basket. Want to avoid 500 calories' worth of blood sugar–raising refined carbs and artery-blocking saturated fat? Politely ask the server to take that bread-and-butter basket back to the kitchen. (If that's too drastic, take *one* piece first—but just one.)

Start with water or unsweetened iced tea. After that, limit yourself to one cocktail or glass of wine or beer and have it with or after your meal. For many people, alcohol triggers extra nibbling.

Ask lots of questions. Is the chicken in the salad grilled or battered and fried? What's in the mashed potatoes? Can you get two veggies instead of the fries and coleslaw or a small fruit salad instead of the mountain of hash browns? Can the fish be broiled? Most restaurants will be happy to accommodate you; if there's a small extra charge for some substitutions, it's usually worth it.

Always ask for sauces and dressings on the side. You don't need 4 ounces of creamy dressing on your salad. In fact, when possible, choose dressings and sauces made with good fats such as olive oil instead of with cream and butter. Spoon a little over your food or dip the tines of your fork in the sauce before spearing a forkful of food. Plan to leave most of the dressing or sauce uneaten. After all, it's just for flavor.

Fast Food Survival Guide

Amazing facts: Where can you find a side salad packed with veggies, or a yogurt-and-fruit parfait? At a fast-food drive-through. Where can you order a 600-calorie cup of coffee and a sandwich that delivers as many calories and as much fat as *three* McDonald's Quarter Pounders? In the food court of your local shopping mall, sports arena, or airport.

Navigating the nutritional gold mines—and land mines—of these everyday eateries requires a smart plan of attack. Here's how to rein in the calories, fat, and salt—and get a healthy dose of fruit, veggies, lean protein, and low-fat dairy at the same time.

Fast food: Order the smallest burger, grilled chicken (no sauce), or a salad that contains little or no cheese (ask for packets of fat-free dressing). Sip water, unsweetened tea, low-fat milk, or a diet soft drink. If you've just gotta have fries, stick with the smallest size. Look for these gems: Veggie burgers, side salads, sliced fruit, and yogurt.

Food court: Order salads with fat-free dressing and no cheese; made-to-order turkey sandwiches on whole wheat with lettuce, tomato, and plain mustard; small burgers; or grilled chicken. Drink water, a diet soft drink, unsweetened tea, or regular coffee. If you order a cappuccino or latte, ask for fat-free milk. Skip sweet coffee drinks and oversize mall desserts, such as cookies and cinnamon buns.

Choose a veggie starter. A simple salad or vegetable plate is a heart-smart alternative to all those high-fat, high-calorie, high-sodium appetizers, such as fried cheese, nachos, Buffalo wings, or cheese-drenched potato skins.

Outsmart super-size portions. Did you know that china manufacturers have resized their tableware to accommodate restaurant portions that are now two to seven times bigger than before? Even the healthiest menu choice can become a heart attacker in those quantities! Learn how to downsize larger-than-life servings.

- Order from the left side of the menu. Most appetizers are the perfect size for a meal. Have one protein-based appetizer as your main dish and one vegetable-based selection as your side dish. Be sure to tell the server that these are your meal and should be brought when the other guests' entrées arrive.

- Ask the server to box half your entrée before serving it or ask for a take-home box when your meal arrives, then immediately put half inside. Out of sight, out of mouth.

- Share. Order a small salad for yourself, then split an entrée with a companion.

- Be a kid again. While sit-down restaurants usually prohibit it, fast-food restaurants don't care if grown-ups order kids' meals for themselves. Today, a kids' meal at major fast-food chains is often the size an adult portion was 20 years ago. A hamburger, small fries, and low-fat milk or orange juice are surprisingly filling and contain a fraction of the calories of "super" meals. They're not particularly nutritious, but for those who can't break their fast-food habit, they're a good compromise.

Deadly Secrets of the Restaurant Trade

How do restaurants make their food taste so good? You probably don't want to know—but deep down, you already have it figured out.

Butter: In the soup. In the sauce. On the meat. On the vegetables. Using butter is the easiest, quickest way to make things taste rich and wonderful (the basic recipe for Buffalo-style hot wing sauce? Equal parts butter and pepper sauce). Most restaurants go through huge amounts; never mind that it's pure saturated fat.

Oil: Another way to make foods taste richer is to use lots of oil. Sometimes it's olive oil, and sometimes it's more exotic nut oils for unique flavor. At lower-grade restaurants, it's old-fashioned vegetable oil. (Take note of what collects on the bottom of the container the next time you get takeout Chinese or Mexican.) This is also why fried foods taste good: They're sponges for the oil they're cooked in.

Animal fat: The next time you see restaurant steaks or hamburgers described as juicy, remember: Meat "juices" are mostly melted fat. Sauces made "au jus" are often extremely calorie dense and unhealthy for your heart.

Salt: Cook at home, and you shake a little salt in as you go. At a restaurant, it's *poured* in to extract maximum flavor.

Sweeteners: Ever have a side dish of vegetables that tasted sweeter than the dessert that followed the meal? That's because of all the added sugar.

The 30-Minutes-A-Day Restaurant Guide

Here's how to spot the healthy gems hiding on some typical menus.

CHINESE

Go for: Stir-fried (request little or no oil) or steamed dishes with lots of vegetables, steamed rice, or poached fish, or entrées that contain chicken, seafood, or just vegetables. Ask for brown rice, not white. Look for these Chinese words: *jum* (poached), *chu* (boiled), and *kow* (roasted).

Avoid: Fried stuff such as crispy wonton appetizers, egg or spring rolls, fried rice, and shrimp toast. Limit sodium by asking for low-sodium soy sauce and no monosodium glutamate (MSG) in your food.

ITALIAN

Go for: Red, clam, or noncreamy seafood sauces and grilled or roasted chicken or fish.

Avoid: Entrées smothered in cream and butter sauces, such as fettuccine Alfredo; anything topped with carbonara or served "parmigiana" (with melted cheese); and pasta stuffed with cheese or fatty meat.

MEXICAN

Go for: Fajitas—you build them yourself, piling grilled veggies and chicken, shrimp, or beef on a flour tortilla. Add lettuce, tomato, and peppers; skip or limit the shredded cheese and guacamole (yes, avocado is packed with good fat, but many commercial varieties are also full of added saturated fat). Also good: simple burritos and soft tacos, grilled chicken and fish, and black beans. The best sauces to choose are salsa and pico de gallo.

Avoid: Fat-drenched refried beans, fried items such as chimichangas, and cheese-covered nachos and entrées.

JAPANESE

Go for: Sushi and sashimi, soba or udon noodles, yakitori (chicken teriyaki), shumai (steamed dumplings), tofu, sukiyaki and kayaku goban (vegetables and rice).

Avoid: Shrimp or vegetable tempura, chicken katsu, tonkatsu (fried pork), shrimp agemono, and fried tofu (bean curd).

UPSCALE AMERICAN CAFÉ

Go for: Seafood broiled with lemon and herbs, pan-roasted meats, interesting vegetable dishes, and whole-meal salads built on mixed greens but with dressing on the side. Choose broth-based, not creamy, soups.

Avoid: Items made with cheese, fatty meats, cream, and butter.

BREAKFAST HOUSES

Go for: Whole wheat pancakes, topped with fruit; vegetable-filled omelets; whole wheat or rye toast with jam; one- or two-egg dishes (the standard omelet in some restaurants now has four eggs!); Canadian bacon; lots of fruit; low-fat cottage cheese; grill-top home fries; granola with low-fat milk; orange juice.

Avoid: Butter (many restaurants use tons of it on eggs, toast, pancakes, and hash browns); whipped cream on your waffles or pancakes; regular bacon or sausage; cream in your coffee; white bread toast; waffles or pancakes made with bleached, refined flour.

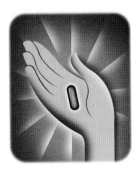

Supplement Power

YOU'LL EAT PLENTY of heart-nurturing, nutrient-packed food on the 30-Minutes-A-Day Eating Plan—and further strengthen and pamper your ticker with exercise, stress reduction, and even joy and friendship. Is there any reason to add supplements? Until recently, the answer from the medical establishment would have been an emphatic "no." Now, though, there's compelling evidence that vitamins, minerals, and other safe, well-chosen nutritional supplements repair and protect your heart in ways that go beyond a health-conscious lifestyle. Adding them to your plan could add healthy years to your life.

Why? Supplements fill gaps created by less-than-perfect eating habits and metabolic changes that happen naturally with age. They shore up deficiencies that are unintentional "side effects" of other healthy choices (a prime example: If you avoid the sun to cut skin cancer risk, your body may be making less vitamin D than you need). Supplements aren't a substitute for healthy living. Their job is to top off your tank with the natural tools your heart needs for optimal health—such as multivitamins, fish oil, soluble fiber, and coenzyme Q_{10}—and to add a few higher-tech helpers, such as low-dose aspirin, cholesterol-blocking phytosterols, and even prescription-strength niacin, for more protection against heart attack and heart failure.

As you'll see on page 126, we recommend you take four supplements daily, and talk to your doctor about four others. Is eight pills a day excessive? You be the final judge. But we believe the science behind our recommended supplements is so compelling that few doctors would argue against them.

1 MULTIVITAMINS The Cornerstone of the Plan

The American Medical Association (AMA) made headlines two years ago when, for the first time, it advised all adults to take daily multivitamins to help prevent heart disease, cancer, and osteoporosis. Until then, the AMA had maintained that unless you were pregnant or chronically ill, you could get the nutrients you needed from food. Despite that advice, though, just one in three of us pop a daily multivitamin today. Here's why you should.

✓ **Heart benefits:** Taking a multi cuts the risk of cardiovascular disease by 24 percent and slashes heart attack risk by 22 percent for men and 33 percent for women.

✓ **How it works:**

• **Lowers homocysteine.** The B vitamins in a multi can cut homocysteine levels by a whopping 32 percent, report Harvard researchers, whose review of hundreds of vitamin studies prompted the AMA to finally recommend multivitamins for everyone.

Homocysteine, an amino acid produced when your body breaks down protein, is an emerging risk factor for heart disease and stroke. Your body needs the "three Bs"—vitamins B_6 and B_{12} and folate (or folic acid, the supplement form)—to convert homocysteine into a form that cells can use to build new proteins. Otherwise, homocysteine levels rise, and so does heart risk. As we age, our bodies absorb less and less of the B vitamins in food, but luckily, the Bs in supplements are well absorbed.

• **Cools off chronic inflammation.** A daily multi lowered levels of C-reactive protein, a sign of heart-threatening inflammation, by 32 percent in a study at the Cooper Institute in Dallas. And in research from Duke University Medical Center, a multi cut levels of another dangerous inflammatory chemical interleukin-6.

• **Protects "bad" LDL cholesterol against artery-damaging free radicals.** The Cooper Institute's vitamin research also revealed that getting into the multivitamin habit helps shield LDLs from oxidation, a key step in the process that pumps gunky plaque into artery walls. Multis reduced LDL damage by 17 percent in one study.

• **Provides protective vitamin D.** Getting regular vitamin D supplements reduced heart disease deaths by 31 percent in a huge study of 10,000 women conducted at the University of California, San Francisco. Among other duties, vitamin D helps the body absorb and hold on to calcium, which is important for healthy blood pressure. It may also guard against the buildup of artery-hardening calcium deposits, and research from Belgium suggests that D cools off body-wide inflammation. Your body produces D naturally when exposed to sunshine, but if you shun the sun or live in the northern half of the United States, you probably don't get enough sun exposure to make enough of the vitamin.

✓ **Best kind to buy:** Not necessarily the most expensive multi on the rack—plenty of store brands offer the same complete range of vitamins and minerals, at the right doses, for far less money. (For the right combination and dose of micronutrients, see "Pick the Perfect Multivitamin" on page 122.)

✓ **Best dose:** One per day.

✓ **When to take it:** With food for best absorption.

✓ **Side effects:** Mild nausea. If this happens, take your multi with a meal.

✓ **Cautions:** Take only the recommended dose.

✓ **Smart tip:** Take your multi with a full glass of water for better absorption.

Pick the Perfect Multivitamin

Think of your multivitamin as an insurance policy—not a replacement for a healthy diet. Look for these levels of important nutrients.

100 Percent of the Big Nine: Make sure your multivitamin has 100 percent of the Daily Value (DV) for thiamin (vitamin B_1); riboflavin (vitamin B_2); niacin (vitamin B_3); folic acid; and vitamins B_6, B_{12}, C, D, and E.

Less Than 2,500 IU of Retinol-Based Vitamin A: Getting more than 5,000 IU of vitamin A daily from retinol may increase your osteoporosis risk. Look for supplements containing no more than 2,500 IU of vitamin A or, if those aren't available, supplements with 5,000 IU, of which at least 50 percent comes from beta-carotene.

No More Than 100 Percent of Minerals: You don't need more than 100 percent of the DV for chromium, copper, iodine, manganese, molybdenum, and zinc, and most people get plenty of chloride, magnesium, phosphorus, and potassium from a healthy diet. Trace ele-ments, such as boron, nickel, silicon, tin, and vanadium, aren't necessary, since they may not even be required by humans.

Vitamin K: At Least 20 Micrograms: Few multivitamins come close to supplying 100 percent of the recommended daily intake of vitamin K (90 to 120 micrograms). Plan to make up the difference with broccoli and green leafy veggies. (If you take a blood-thinning drug, talk to your doc first.)

Iron: Your Age and Sex Matter: Premenopausal women should look for 18 milligrams of iron in a multi. Men and postmenopausal women should look for supplements without iron.

Final Note: Some multivitamin makers sell premium versions that include "proprietary blends" of herbs, minerals, extracts, and amino acids, often with a targeted health goal. Be cautious with these. While many of the individual ingredients may have research that supports them, no one has looked at the efficacy of these blends. You might be paying extra money for a mix of ingredients of little or no value.

The 30-Minutes-A-Day Healthy Heart Supplement Plan

For maximum heart protection, we urge you to take the first four supplements every day and consult your doctor about whether you should include any of the following four.

SUPPLEMENT	DAILY DOSE	NOTES
WE RECOMMEND:		
Multivitamin	1	—
Calcium	1,000–1,200 mg	—
Fish oil	1–2 g omega-3s	—
Soluble fiber	7–10 g	—
ALSO CONSIDER:		
Aspirin	81 mg (one low-dose aspirin)	Talk to your doctor first
Coenzyme Q_{10}	100 mg	For hypertension and for statin users
Phytosterols	2 g	Only if cholesterol is elevated
Niacin	500–1,000 mg	Prescription-strength only; talk to your doctor

2 FISH OIL Like Eating Salmon Every Day

Your heart loves a good fish dinner: Research suggests that even two fish meals a week could cut heart attack risk by 25 to 50 percent or more. The catch: The fish has to be rich in two heart-friendly omega-3 fatty acids—eicosapentaenoic acid (EPA) and docosahexaenoic acid (DHA)—and most of us don't get enough of this good stuff. Can fish oil in capsules fill the gap? Studies show that it cuts risk of a second heart attack by 20 percent. The American Heart Association suggests that heart patients who don't eat fish regularly should add daily fish-oil capsules; we think a daily dose of this natural fat is good for nearly everybody.

✓**Heart benefits:** Omega-3 fatty acids, found in fish-oil capsules as well as in fatty fish like salmon and mackerel, can cut heart attack risk by a whopping 73 percent when consumed daily as part of a diet packed with fruits, veggies, and whole grains and low in saturated fat. Omega-3s also cut triglyceride levels up to 30 to 40 percent.

✓**How it works:**
• **Stabilizes dangerous artery plaque.** Researchers at the University of Southampton asked 178 people awaiting artery-clearing surgery to take fish oil, sunflower oil, or placebos (dummy capsules) every day for up to six months before their operations. After surgery, the researchers found evidence that the fish-oil group's plaque was far less likely to rupture and cause heart-threatening blood clots.

• **Lowers triglycerides.** Triglyceride levels rise after eating a fatty meal—a fact that may explain higher heart attack rates following a big breakfast, lunch, or dinner. In a University of Missouri study, men who took fish-oil supplements had triglyceride levels that were 35 to 50 percent lower than normal after eating big meals—a decline that could save your life. Researchers speculate that fish oil helps muscle cells break down triglycerides more efficiently, vacuuming them out of the bloodstream.

• **Keeps hearts on the beat.** Wildly irregular heartbeats (arrhythmias) can trigger sudden cardiac death. In a study published in the *Lancet*, British researchers found that fish oil significantly protected the hearts of women and men who wore pacemakers to guard against heartbeat irregularities. When the scientists tried to induce arrhythmias in the volunteers, 7 of 10 had out-of-rhythm beats before receiving fish oil; after taking it, only 2 did.

✓**Best kind to buy:** Two tests of fish-oil supplements—one by *Consumer Reports,* the other by ConsumerLab.com—found no significant amounts of mercury in topselling brands. That means you don't have to pay extra for pharmaceutical-grade fish oil; the stuff in the drugstore is fine.

✓**Best dose:** Experts suggest getting a total of 1 to 2 grams, combined, of EPA and DHA. How many capsules is that? Read labels; the dose varies by brand.

✓**When to take it:** With food.

✓**Side effects:** Fishy burps, mild nausea, and bloating.

✓**Caution:** Fish oil's anticlotting powers could be dangerous for people with bleeding disorders and those who take anticoagulant medications such as warfarin (Coumadin). Talk to your doctor before starting to take fish-oil supplements.

✓**Smart tip:** Refrigerate the capsules or take them on a full stomach to eliminate fishy burps.

3 SOLUBLE FIBER Cholesterol-Lowering Powerhouse

Oatmeal and beans, barley and oranges, grapefruit and strawberries are all rich in soluble fiber—an indigestible carbohydrate that forms a thick, cholesterol-trapping gel in your digestive system. You need at least 8 grams a day—and more like 10 to 25 grams if you have elevated cholesterol—yet most of us take in barely 4 grams daily (about the amount in a bowl of oatmeal and a handful of strawberries).

That's why the 30-Minutes-A-Day Plan includes a soluble fiber supplement—not as a substitute for fiber-rich grains and produce, but because getting extra soluble fiber is the safest, most powerful drug-free way to knock your cholesterol down a notch. In fact, top fiber researchers say that about 15 percent of the people whose doctors recommend statin drugs to lower slightly elevated cholesterol could get the job done with a healthier diet and a soluble fiber supplement.

✓ **Heart benefits:** Soluble fiber cuts total cholesterol by 7 percent and LDL cholesterol by 5 percent, which translates into a 10 to 15 percent reduction in heart disease risk. Fiber supplements are best for people who want to prevent heart problems; if you have known heart disease, don't use them in place of recommended drug therapy.

✓ **How it works:** Soluble fiber forms a thick gel that moves slowly through your intestines, snagging cholesterol-packed bile acids and ushering them out of the body. Your liver manufactures bile acids to help break down fats for digestion. Usually, 95 percent of the cholesterol in these acids is reabsorbed, but soluble fiber drags them out of the body. This forces the liver to draw cholesterol from the bloodstream to manufacture more bile acids. The bottom line: Your cholesterol levels drop.

✓ **Best kind to buy:** Base your decision on your personal taste and convenience. Fiber supplements come as flavored powders that you mix with water, as capsules, and even as wafers. Supplements can be made from ground psyllium seed (the most extensively researched fiber supplement for cutting cholesterol), from beta-glucan (the same fiber that's in oatmeal), and from fibers called inulin, methylcellulose, and polycarbophil.

✓ **Best dose:** Aim for 7 to 10 grams of soluble fiber from supplements daily. Check the product you choose; each supplement has a different fiber content.

✓ **When to take it:** Take half in the morning and the other half sometime in the evening.

✓ **Side effects:** A bloated feeling, gas, and constipation.

✓ **Caution:** Discuss fiber supplements with your physician first if you have a bowel obstruction, an ulcer, or chronic constipation. In rare cases, psyllium can cause an allergic reaction. Seek emergency medical help if you develop fast or irregular breathing, a skin rash, hives, or itching after taking a psyllium product.

✓ **Smart tip:** If you take a prescription drug, take your fiber supplement at least 2 hours before or after. Always take a fiber supplement as directed (in other words, a double dose is not a good idea), with at least one 8-ounce glass of water; two glasses are even better. And if you're new to fiber supplements, go slowly. For the first week, take just one dose per day, then work up to your goal over a month or so to avoid discomfort.

4 PHYTOSTEROLS A New Way to Block Bad LDLs

Found naturally in soybeans, rice bran, and wheat germ, plant sterols and stanols—known collectively as phytosterols—block the absorption of cholesterol from the food you eat. Now these ingenious substances are available in capsules and in special cholesterol-lowering margarines. Even the National Institutes of Health recommends two helpings per day to help lower cholesterol.

✓ **Heart benefits:** A daily phytosterol supplement can lower your LDL cholesterol levels by 13 to 21 mg/dl—a reduction that cuts heart risk by up to 21 percent.

✓ **How they work:** The chemical structure of phytosterols is almost identical to that of cholesterol. In your intestines, phytosterols bind with molecules that normally carry cholesterol into the bloodstream. The result: "Unwanted" cholesterol is eliminated during bowel movements.

✓ **Best kind to buy:** Look for sterols and stanols in cholesterol-lowering margarines, such as Benecol and Take Control, and as capsules.

✓ **Best dose:** Get 2 to 3 grams a day. That's 2 to 3 tablespoons of margarine; pill doses vary by brand.

✓ **When to take it:** With meals to block dietary cholesterol absorption. Have a tablespoon of margarine on your morning toast and another with lunch, dinner, or a snack.

✓ **Side effects:** None when you use the recommended amount.

✓ **Caution:** Some research suggests that phytosterols can slightly reduce levels of fat-soluble vitamins, like beta-carotene, so get an extra serving of beta-carotene-rich foods (such as carrots, sweet potatoes, and yellow squash) every day. For better absorption, eat them when you're not using phytosterol margarine or a supplement.

✓ **Smart tip:** Switching from a smidgen of regular margarine on your morning toast to cholesterol-lowering margarine? You may need a bigger portion than you're accustomed to. Use a measuring spoon at first to see what a 1-tablespoon portion looks like.

Antioxidant Supplements: Extra Protection or Duds?

Antioxidant pills sound good in theory. For years, experts have recommended getting megadoses of vitamin E and beta-carotene to help protect your heart. The reasoning made sense, since antioxidants neutralize plaque-promoting free radicals—destructive particles released naturally when you breathe, digest your breakfast, or are exposed to toxins such as cigarette smoke. Getting extra antioxidants *should* equal extra protection.

For reasons the experts don't fully understand, however, pills don't help. Taking antioxidant vitamins is at best a waste of money; at worst, it may actually raise your risk of a deadly heart attack. When scientists at the Cleveland Clinic in Ohio examined seven big studies on vitamin E and eight large studies on beta-carotene and heart health, they concluded that E offered no protection. Even more troubling: Beta-carotene raised the risk of death from cardiovascular disease.

The bottom line: Get your vitamin E from three servings of whole grains and wheat germ per day, and fill up on beta-carotene (and hundreds of other antioxidants) by loading your plate with fruits and veggies.

5 COENZYME Q₁₀ Power Up Your Heart Muscle

Dubbed "vitamin Q_{10}" and even "ubiquinone" because it's found everywhere in the body (ubiquitous), coenzyme Q_{10} (CoQ_{10}) boosts the effectiveness of enzymes that help cells produce energy. Getting sufficient CoQ_{10} ensures that heart-muscle cells will pump efficiently; it can also cut symptoms of heart failure and shield cells from free radical damage.

✓ **Heart benefits:** Numerous studies—some mentioned below—show that CoQ_{10} has many heart benefits. Many are linked to its antioxidant properties: by removing free radicals from the bloodstream, it helps lead to lower blood pressure and less oxidative stress.

✓ **How it works:**

• Helps damaged heart muscle grow stronger. In the 1950s, researchers first noticed that people with heart disease are low in CoQ_{10}. Experts suspect it helps mitochondria, the tiny power plants inside your cells, produce energy. In one 12-month study of 2,500 people with heart failure, 80 percent of those who took CoQ_{10} noticed improvement in their symptoms—they retained less fluid and had less shortness of breath, and they slept better. (Not all studies have shown a benefit, however.)

• Controls blood pressure. Up to one-third of people with high blood pressure may have low levels of CoQ_{10}. When researchers from the Department of Veterans Affairs Medical Center in Boise, Idaho, gave CoQ_{10} supplements to 83 people with high blood pressure, 55 percent saw their levels drop—some by more than 17 points. The mechanism? Experts think CoQ_{10} calms hypertension by reducing free radical damage inside arteries.

• Offsets statin problems. Some cardiologists recommend adding CoQ_{10} if you take a statin drug because these drugs block production of CoQ_{10} in the liver—a side effect that some experts would like to see listed as a warning on the drugs' labels.

✓ **Best kind to take:** For best absorption, look for capsules or tablets with CoQ_{10} in an oil base.

✓ **Dose:** 100 milligrams per day.

✓ **When to take it:** With a meal. CoQ_{10} is fat soluble, so your body will absorb much more if you take it with a fat-containing food, such as the oil in salad dressing.

✓ **Side effects:** Usually none. Very rarely, it can cause mild insomnia, stomach upset, or loss of appetite.

✓ **Caution:** May reduce the effectiveness of blood-thinning medicines such as warfarin.

✓ **Smart tip:** If you're being treated for high blood pressure or heart failure, discuss CoQ_{10} with your doctor; it's not a substitute for medication.

Hawthorn: A Berry Good "Heart Vitamin"

Hawthorn berry extract is an age-old heart tonic that has new science to back it up. In the *Journal of Family Practice*, researchers noted that this herbal extract is a good add-on therapy for people with heart failure because it seems to improve blood flow to the heart and help stabilize out-of-rhythm heartbeats. Hawthorn isn't a substitute for heart medication or for any of the other supplements in this chapter, but as an added therapy, it just may do your heart some good. The best dose? Follow the label directions.

6 ASPIRIN Stop That Clot

Recently, heart experts have realized that aspirin's pain-soothing, inflammation-cooling active ingredient—acetylsalicylic acid—is also a potent heart protector that works by cutting clot risk.

✓ **Heart benefits:** A daily low-dose aspirin can cut your risk of a heart attack by 33 percent. The U.S. Preventive Services Task Force recommends daily aspirin for heart health for men over 40; postmenopausal women; and younger people with any cardiovascular disease history or risk factors, such as smoking, high blood pressure, high cholesterol, diabetes, or a sedentary lifestyle. Despite this, among people who *should* take daily aspirin, just 45 percent of women and 58 percent of men do.

✓ **How it works:** Aspirin inhibits the clumping action of blood platelets, cells responsible for the dangerous or even deadly blood clots that cause a heart attack or ischemic stroke. Experts aren't sure whether it works as an anti-inflammatory at low doses.

✓ **Best dose:** Talk to your doctor. Generally, the recommended dose is 81 milligrams per day. Higher doses don't offer more protection; in fact, doses over 100 milligrams a day can double your risk of gastrointestinal (GI) bleeding.

✓ **When to take it:** With a meal to cut GI bleeding risk.

✓ **Best kind to buy:** Low-dose or "baby" aspirin. Be sure that the dose is less than 100 milligrams.

✓ **Side effects:** In some people, aspirin can cause stomach bleeding or kidney failure or raise the risk of a less common type of stroke called hemorrhagic stroke.

911 for Heart Attack: Call on Aspirin

If you or someone you're with has sudden heart attack symptoms, thoroughly chewing and swallowing one regular-strength aspirin tablet immediately while you're waiting for the ambulance to arrive can be a lifesaver. Chewing delivers aspirin's clot-stopping power to the bloodstream in just 5 minutes; in contrast, swallowing the aspirin whole delays the clot stoppers for 12 crucial minutes.

✓ **Caution:** If you take the pain reliever ibuprofen, wait 2 hours before taking aspirin: ibuprofen can interfere with aspirin's heart-protective powers, although researchers aren't sure why. If you take ibuprofen regularly and want to add aspirin to your heart-smart regimen, talk to your doctor about switching to an alternative painkiller such as a COX-2 inhibitor, which may not interfere with aspirin.

✓ **Smart tip:** For genetic reasons, 20 to 35 percent of aspirin users may be resistant to its anticlotting effects; ask your doctor about a blood test called VerifyNow Aspirin that checks whether the active ingredient in aspirin inhibits platelet aggregation in your blood. If you're resistant and at high risk for heart disease, consider a prescription anticlotting drug called clopidogrel (Plavix).

How is it that exercise became so scientific and scary? We say, just get up and move! Next to a healthy diet, nothing is better for your heart than being on your feet.

Rise Up Against Sitting Disease

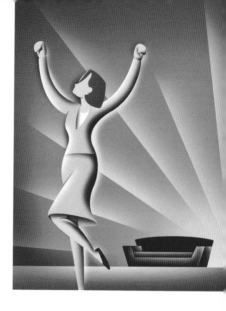

ARE YOU SITTING down? If you are, you've got plenty of company. You are engaged in an *un*-activity that the typical American now spends an amazing amount of time doing. No one keeps accurate statistics on our cumulative sitting time, but the available data reveal that the average American is seated for 12 to 14 hours each day: behind the wheel of a car (1 to 2 hours); watching television (3 hours); and parked behind a desk, working either on the job or at home (7 to 9 hours). Add an hour of sitting at mealtimes and 7 hours of shut-eye, and you're looking at an astonishing 19 to 22 hours of almost complete downtime.

For many, the numbers are worse. Think about the most sedentary people you know. Can you honestly say they are on their feet for 3 hours a day? Probably not. We would guess that there are millions of Americans who spend as little as an hour being up and moving briskly during a typical day.

Ironically, our ancestors would have been thrilled with this chair-centric lifestyle. They toiled from sunrise to sunset just to have a meal to sit down to at the end of the day. Today, we barely budge from our seats to get breakfast. Through the genius of remote controls, dishwashers, drive-thrus, automatic windows, e-mail, and Internet shopping, we've engineered physical activity almost completely out of our lives—so much so that some experts estimate that we burn up to 700 fewer calories each day than we did just 30 years ago. That adds up to well over a pound a week. "Consider the energy savings of a single e-mail," says Joyce A. Hanna, associate director of the Health Improvement Program at Stanford University. "If you were to walk across the building and back to talk to someone instead of spending the same 2 minutes sending an e-mail, you could save 11 pounds over 10 years." And that's just one e-mail per day!

Because our modern lives require so little physical labor, our only source of exercise is physical fun such as walking, gardening, and sports, but woefully few of us find time for that, either. National surveys report that one-quarter of adults—and a full one-third of women—do absolutely no leisure-time physical activities. Another third don't do enough for meaningful health benefits. Given these stats, it's hardly a coincidence that two-thirds of the population now tip their bathroom scales into the danger zone; that 25 to 30 percent of us have high blood pressure; and that a quarter of all deaths each year are the direct result of chronic illnesses linked to sedentary living.

Vitamin X for a Healthy Heart

Just as we restore lost vitamins and minerals to white bread and refined cereal, we must fortify our lives with the activity we've removed. Consider it your daily dose of vitamin X (for exercise), which is every bit as essential for heart health as the nutrients you swallow in your morning supplements.

What's so important about exercise? When you walk, pull dandelions, or swing a 5-iron, your heart grows stronger, so it can pump more blood with every beat and perform work with less stress and strain. Regular daily exercise also fends off heart disease on a number of specific fronts.

🩶 It brings down blood pressure

Physical activity is like a Roto-Rooter for your

Time Investment

Your goal is to sit less for 1 hour a day (including the time you spend with the easy exercise plans outlined in this section). That doesn't mean you have to block out a big chunk of your daily schedule or add anything to your to-do list, although you can if you like. By swapping sedentary moments for moments in motion, you'll move more, feel better, and live longer.

arteries, flushing them clean and keeping them clear and supple. In a recent study of more than 500 men and women ages 40 to 60, researchers found that physical activity is inversely related to the progressive buildup of plaque in the carotid arteries. Even people who played golf or gardened just a day or two a week had clearer arteries than those who did no leisure-time activity.

🩶 It burns off blood sugar

Studies have shown that a single bout of exercise improves blood sugar metabolism immediately and for up to 24 hours afterward. A recent Duke University study revealed that long-term, regular exercise can improve your insulin sensitivity (how efficiently your body stimulates glucose, or blood sugar, metabolism) by about 24 percent.

🩶 It controls weight

Exercise burns calories so you lose, or at least don't gain, weight. But even if you can't shed all those stubborn pounds, you'll reap big benefits. Cardiologists recently determined in a study that among people whose BMI averaged 41 (that's morbidly obese), those who lost just 7 percent of their body weight through regular exercise regained healthy blood pressure and triglyceride levels, and the inflammation in their arteries dropped by between a quarter and a third, even though their BMI still averaged 38. Numerous studies have confirmed that you don't need to be skinny to be physically fit.

🤍 It cuts cholesterol

It's well known that exercise helps lower cholesterol through weight loss. A study from Duke University also showed that physical activity, even without weight loss, actually changes the structure of protein particles that carry cholesterol, making it less able to cause artery damage and heart disease.

🤍 It banks more beats

Every 60 seconds, the average couch potato's heart beats 70 to 75 times—more than a beat per second. An active person's heart, on the other hand, is so strong that it can pump the same amount of blood in only 50 beats. That's 36,000 fewer beats every day and 13 *million* fewer by the end of just one year. Common sense says that the less strenuously your engine has to work, the longer it will chug along trouble-free.

🤍 It lifts stress and sadness

Studies show that exercise can work as well as drugs to alleviate depression and reduce stress. The Mayo Clinic recently reported that just 10 minutes of moderate-intensity exercise can enhance your mood—a potential lifesaver for people with heart disease. In a recent study of more than 2,000 men and women who had had heart attacks, those who were depressed or socially isolated were more than twice as

Then and Now

Yes, we all understand that life is much easier today than it was before cars and electricity, but few of us ponder the details. Here are some specifics of why sitting disease is such a modern affair.

TASK	NOW	THEN
Get fuel for transportation	Lower car window at gas station, ask for unleaded.	Go to barn daily, feed horse, clean stall.
Get fuel for heat	Pay monthly electric, gas, or heating-oil bill.	Spend hours a day chopping and stacking wood.
Take a bath	Turn faucet.	Fetch water from river or pump, make fire, heat water, pour into tub.
Go to town	Get into car and drive.	Walk, ride horse, or attach horse to carriage.
Wash clothes	Put in washing machine.	Fetch and boil water, scrub each piece by hand.
Dry clothes	Put in dryer.	Hang ropes outside, hang each piece.
Have a steak	Outback, anyone?	Elsie, you were a good cow, but...
Say hi to Aunt Mae	Hmmm, should I e-mail or call today?	Write letter, walk to post office.
Get a new chair	"Honey, I'm going to IKEA."	"Honey, I'm going to chop down a tree."
Get butter for bread	Retrieve from refrigerator door.	Milk cow, churn cream.
Evening routine	Watch TV, snack.	Sleep; that's what you do when the sun is down.
Early-morning routine	Sleep, shower, make coffee, commute.	Work; that's what you do when the sun is up.

likely to die of second heart attacks if they didn't exercise.

💜 *It breaks bad habits*

Moving your behind helps you kick butts. In a study of 280 women, researchers at Brown University found that women who quit smoking and started exercising were twice as likely to stay smoke-free—and gained half as much weight—as women who quit without exercising.

Time *Is* on Your Side

The number one excuse people give for not exercising is, you guessed it, no time. But closer inspection reveals that Americans actually have more—that's right, *more*—free time than ever. We've just been using it sitting down—with a bag of chips—in front of the television.

Studies show that we have almost 5 hours more free time per week than we did in the 1960s. It only *feels* like less because we cram more tasks into each second while we're on the job. "Thanks" to technology, we can skim the news, call a friend, write a report, plan our next vacation, and buy Bruce Springsteen's new album in less than an hour—without leaving our chairs. When we get home, we feel so frazzled, so mentally exhausted, that we plop down and watch TV for as much as 5-*plus* hours a day (there goes that free time), according to a study from Ball State University, where researchers actually sat in people's homes and recorded their viewing habits. The catch: Instead of energizing us as exercise would, TV leaves us even more lifeless.

That may explain why our other leisure-time activities are growing more leisurely as well. A recent poll of more than 1,000 men and women found that only 29 percent of Americans' current favorite pastimes involve any physical activity, down from 38 percent just 10 years ago. Reading, watching TV, and spending time with family—mostly sitting and eating—top the list of ways we like

Doing It Yourself

Timesaving devices may save us minutes, but they can literally take years off our lives by stealing opportunities to keep our bodies strong and fit. Use a little muscle instead of a machine with these heart-healthy swaps.

INSTEAD OF...	GET ACTIVE BY...
Hiring a full-time cleaning service	Doing 1 hour of your own vacuuming and dusting once a week
Driving to the carwash	Washing and waxing your own car once a month
Internet shopping	Hitting your favorite shopping district for 90 minutes of brisk buying once a month
Activating the electric fence	Walking Rover around the block each day
Leaving yard work to the lawn service	Mowing the lawn or trimming the bushes for 1 hour each week
Driving to the corner store	Walking or taking your bike
Blowing leaves	Raking them
Using the dishwasher	Hand washing dishes once or twice a week
Letting helping hands shoulder the load	Carrying and unloading your own groceries

to spend our time, while past favorites such as swimming, walking, running, and gardening have fallen out of favor. We don't even fish or bowl as much as we used to.

Of all this inactivity, channel surfing is especially hard on your heart. In a six-year study of more than 50,000 women, Harvard researchers found that for every 2 hours a day they spent watching television, the women were 23 percent more likely to be obese and 14 percent more likely to have diabetes. It's a vicious cycle: We sit, we eat, we gain weight, we have no energy—so we keep sitting, and the cycle continues.

We can break the cycle by turning off the television and getting the ball rolling in the opposite direction. The Harvard scientists reported that each hour per day spent fitness walking instead of watching TV can reduce obesity by 24 percent and diabetes by 34 percent. Even puttering around the house for a couple of hours in the evening lowers diabetes risk by 12 percent.

Fitting In Fitness

When you think of exercise, you probably think of structured workouts such as Pilates or running. In fact, aerobics classes and jogging schedules are relatively new and, for many, unnecessary ways to stay fit. You can reap the same rewards with a basic "bottoms-up" approach to fitness—that is, *don't*

sit when you can stand, and don't stand when you can walk. Now, that's a motto to live by!

Small bouts of "lifestyle activity," such as walking around the block after dinner instead of watching a game show or pacing while you talk on the telephone rather than sitting, are by no means intense. Nevertheless, they can be just as good for you as more vigorous exercise, according to research. In a two-year study of more than 230 overweight and inactive men and women, researchers at the Cooper Institute for Aerobics Research in Dallas found that those who sneaked more movement minutes into their days by taking the stairs at the office, parking farther from the door at shopping malls, and pulling weeds around the yard achieved the same improvements in fitness, blood pressure, and body fat as those who went to the gym and exercised vigorously for 20 to 60 minutes five days a week. In a similar study, Johns Hopkins University researchers found that people who added just 30 minutes of lifestyle activity to their days lost almost 10 pounds during the 16-week study period—more than a comparable group who did step aerobics three days a week.

Again, small time investments yield big payoffs. The key is finding active opportunities throughout the day, every day. Once you start looking, you'll be surprised by how many minutes in motion you can rack up.

Most doctors and the government don't consider "sitting" a disease, let alone a

Small time investments yield big pay-offs. The key is finding active opportunities throughout the day, every day.

problem. To them, the notion of "sitting disease" is probably ridiculous! We beg you to think otherwise. In many ways, sedentary living is a much bigger health problem than the more talked-about concerns such as cholesterol and high blood pressure, because if you conquer sitting disease, chances are you'll prevent these other health concerns from ever emerging.

Through the rest of this section, we provide ideas and programs for progressively conquering sitting disease. First, we get you walking, then we get you stretching, then we get you strengthening. All fit in perfectly with the 30-Minutes-A-Day plan; at no point do we ask you to take an hour off to do something you wouldn't otherwise do.

Before we get into more rigorous activity suggestions, though, it's time to get you into an active mindset. By that, we mean pursuing a daily style in which your every choice is the more active alternative. As you go about your day, stand more, walk more, and get outside more!

To get you going, here are some helpful tips that can increase your daily exercise time by 30 to 45 minutes while barely changing your routine.

Take at least two flights a day

Research shows that taking just two flights of stairs a day can add up to a 6-pound weight loss over a year. Regular stair stepping also improves bone density, aerobic fitness, and levels of good cholesterol. Always take the stairs at work and while shopping. If you have stairs at home, make one trip up and down before and after work to be sure you get in at least two flights a day.

Make the pizza

Cooking dinner burns more than twice as many calories as dialing the phone and flipping through a magazine for 20 or 30 minutes as you wait for the chow mein to come. And the food's often better, too. Prep and cook dinner at least one night a week, and preferably five or six nights!

Plan walk 'n' talks

Instead of sitting in a stuffy conference room gnawing stale doughnuts, lead your coworkers outside for roving meetings. Take a small pad and pen to keep notes. Everyone's brain will work better in the fresh air, and you'll have more energy when you return to your office.

Be an active spectator

Your kids' (or grandkids') sports practices and games are terrific opportunities for movement. Pace the sidelines. Walk around the field. Step up and down off the bleachers. The added activity will really give you something to cheer about.

Take the late spots

Five days a week, park in the first spot you see in the lot (usually "reserved" for late-comers). Where it's safe, do the same at malls, restaurants, and other destinations.

Do computer calisthenics

At the top of every hour, straighten and bend each leg 10 times, stand up and rise up and down on your toes 10 times, and stretch your arms to the ceiling before sitting down and resuming work.

Start a walking bus

According to the Centers for Disease Control and Prevention, only 13 percent of kids walk to school—a 66 percent drop from 30 years ago. Start your day off right and help your kids, grandkids, or neighbors' kids fend off future heart disease by starting a "walking school bus": Pick up the children at their homes in the morning and walk with them to school, following a set route. Then do the same in reverse in the afternoon. If the school is too far away, pick a central location, such as a park, where parents can take their kids, and use that as the pickup and drop-off point for your trips. Or caravan by foot to and from a central bus stop.

Pack a ready-to-go bag

Active moments can appear at a moment's notice. Meetings get canceled. Kids run late. Clients are stuck in traffic. Instead of sitting and stewing, strap on your sneaks and take a stroll. Keep a bag packed with sneakers, socks, baby wipes, and a small towel stashed in your car.

Think on your feet

Stand up whenever you need to write a list or jot down notes. It guarantees that you'll get off your seat and stretch your legs a few times a day.

Dial M for "move it"

When the phone rings, stand up, and don't sit down until you're done with the conversation. Walk around the house—or even the yard—to squeeze in extra steps.

Turn ad time into active time

Do chores during the commercial breaks in your favorite TV show or shows. Popping up to do laundry, empty wastebaskets, gather dirty dishes, or wipe countertops can add up to 14 to 24 minutes of activity during an hour-long show, and you'll save hundreds of calories by not snacking instead.

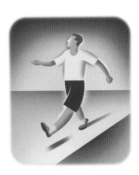

Take Your Heart for a Walk

WALKING CAN SAVE your life. It's a simple, indisputable fact—even if you're just ambling down a city street with shopping bags dangling and kids in tow.

In a landmark Harvard study of nearly 40,000 women over the age of 45, those who walked regularly for exercise—even at a leisurely stroll—for as little as 1 hour per week were *half* as likely to have heart attacks or require surgery for blocked coronary arteries as those who rarely walked.

Putting one foot in front of the other is our most primitive form of locomotion, but this basic skill that you mastered as a youngster can carry your healthy, beating heart well into your nineties and beyond. As proof of the literal power of taking small steps for heart health, researchers with the Honolulu Heart Program observed more than 2,600 men, ages 71 to 93, for a two- to four-year period. At the end of the study, those who walked less than ¼ mile a day—that's two city blocks—were twice as likely to develop heart disease as those who walked at least 1½ miles each day, regardless of pace.

Walking: It's free, simple, and convenient. Anyone can do it almost anywhere. Unfortunately, fewer and fewer of us are doing it anytime or anyplace. Statistics show that the rate of daily walking—for either exercise or transportation—has dropped by 42 percent during the past 20 years. Not coincidentally, the number of obese and overweight Americans has increased by almost 40 percent during the same time period.

Step It Up

Trawl for answers on how much men and women think they walk, and you're likely to reel in a fish story. Sitting disease–plagued Americans notoriously overestimate how much they walk (and underestimate how much they eat—but that's another story).

One way to know for sure is to count your steps—literally. Studies show that the number of steps you take each day has a direct impact on your overall health. And when it comes to weight control, more steps are definitely better. Researchers recently weighed and measured 80 women between the ages of 40 and 66 and then asked them to wear pedometers for one week as they followed their typical work and leisure routines. The investigators found a direct connection between the number of steps taken in a day and the amount of fat stored. On average, those who took the most steps (10,000 or more a day) had only 26 percent body fat and healthy body mass indexes (BMIs), the most popular tool today for tracking the healthiness of your weight. Those who spent more time on their behinds than on their Birkenstocks (stepping out 6,000 or fewer times a day) had an average of 44 percent body fat—well into the obese category—and BMI measurements that clearly put them in the high risk category for heart disease.

Most sedentary folks take only about 3,000 total steps from the time they stumble to the shower in the morning to the time they plod to bed. Although there's no magic number that's right for everyone, and certainly very elderly people may need to take

Walking can carry your healthy, beating heart well into your nineties and beyond.

fewer steps than those in their younger years, experts generally recommend about 10,000 steps as the hallmark of healthy living. As the studies from Harvard and Honolulu clearly illustrate, though, you can get big benefits from even modest step increases. Research shows that for an average person, taking an additional 5,000 to 7,000 steps a day—whether by purposeful "fitness" walking or just pacing while talking on the phone—can reduce the risk of diseases such as cancer, diabetes, osteoporosis, and yes, heart disease. What's more, a recent study from California State University in Long Beach found that the number of steps you take a day has a direct, positive effect on your mood and energy levels—the more, the better.

Of course, no one expects you to walk around all day keeping a mental step count ("8,112, 8,113 . . ."). There are other, much more effective ways to keep track. One is using a simple pedometer. Nicknamed *manpo-kei* (literally, "10,000-steps meter") in Japan, these Post-it–size devices strap onto your waistband and keep a running tally every time you put one foot in front of the other. They sell for about $25 at major sporting goods stores and are becoming increasingly popular among fitness enthusiasts in the United States.

Not a gadget lover? Not a problem. There are many ways to monitor your daily locomotion. One way simply involves mileage. There are approximately 2,000 steps in every mile,

Walk This Way

Walking feels easier when you use good form. Here's what proper walking posture should look like.

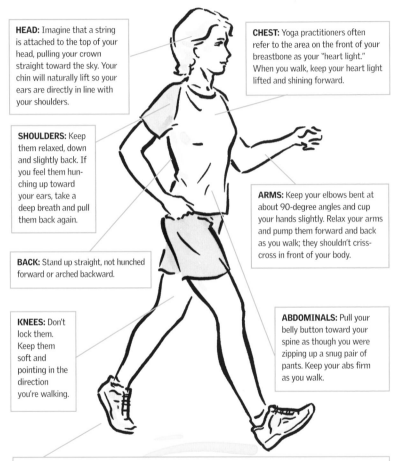

HEAD: Imagine that a string is attached to the top of your head, pulling your crown straight toward the sky. Your chin will naturally lift so your ears are directly in line with your shoulders.

CHEST: Yoga practitioners often refer to the area on the front of your breastbone as your "heart light." When you walk, keep your heart light lifted and shining forward.

SHOULDERS: Keep them relaxed, down and slightly back. If you feel them hunching up toward your ears, take a deep breath and pull them back again.

ARMS: Keep your elbows bent at about 90-degree angles and cup your hands slightly. Relax your arms and pump them forward and back as you walk; they shouldn't criss-cross in front of your body.

BACK: Stand up straight, not hunched forward or arched backward.

KNEES: Don't lock them. Keep them soft and pointing in the direction you're walking.

ABDOMINALS: Pull your belly button toward your spine as though you were zipping up a snug pair of pants. Keep your abs firm as you walk.

FEET: As you take each step, plant your heel, roll onto the ball of your foot, and push off with your toes. Avoid rolling your foot inward or outward. Although you can safely walk short distances in casual dress shoes, wear good walking shoes whenever possible to protect your feet and joints. Your shoes should be designed for walking (or jogging, if walking shoes aren't available) and should feel great right out of the box. For proper fit, be sure there's one finger-width between the end of your longest toe and the front of the inside of the shoe.

so if you know it's ½ mile from your house to the closest mailbox, that's an easy way to keep track. Here are some other guidelines.

Build your blocks

There are about eight city blocks to a mile, so you rack up 250 steps with each block. With the traffic snarls and parking problems that clog most downtown areas, you may find that running errands and grabbing lunch on foot is actually faster—and much better for your bottom-line health—than taking your car.

Watch the clock

Keep track of how many minutes you spend walking, and you'll know whether you accumulated enough steps for the day. As a rule of thumb, you take about 100 steps per minute during everyday ambling. The faster you walk, the more steps you squeeze into every second. Walk as if you were on your way to an appointment, and you'll rack up 120 steps every 60 seconds. Pick up the pace as though you were heading to the bus stop, and you're up to 135 steps a minute. Head out for a power walk—at a pace so brisk that if you went any faster, you'd be jogging—and you'll accumulate 150 steps each minute. To determine how many steps you take with your typical stride, walk as you normally do and count steps for 60 seconds. Repeat three times and calculate the average.

Move to the music

Here's a secret to keep you moving steadily and rhythmically: Most popular music pumps out a predictable number of beats per minute that nicely match a healthy walking pace. So plug in your headset (provided you have either a well-populated, perfectly safe walking environment or a treadmill) and stride to the beat of your favorite tunes. Some classic examples:

- "Kiss" by Prince: 111 bmp (beats per minute)
- "Express Yourself" by Madonna: 115 bpm
- "YMCA" by the Village People: 126 bpm
- "Achy Breaky Heart" by Billy Ray Cyrus: 124 bpm
- "Jump, Jive and Wail" by the Brian Setzer Orchestra: 155 bpm

Factor in non-feet time

If you're already actively swimming or cycling, that counts, too. James O. Hill, Ph.D., author of *The Step Diet*, offers a few "step equivalencies" for popular recreational pastimes.

- 1 minute of cycling = 150 steps
- 1 minute of swimming = 96 steps
- 1 minute of yoga = 50 steps

It's Worth It!

Most of your steps will be woven into the natural fabric of your day, as illustrated in the previous chapter, but we also recommend that you devote 10 to 15 minutes every day to taking your heart for a purposeful, extended walk. By carving out a small chunk of time each day, you're sure to get the minimum dose of weekly walking that's known to protect your heart. You'll also automatically bank about a fifth of your recommended daily steps, so even your most chair-bound, 3,000-step days will include some artery-clearing exercise.

Still not sold on the return from such a short exercise investment? Consider this groundbreaking study from the Harvard School of Public Health. When researchers there examined the activity levels of 7,307 men (average age 66), they found that those who sneaked short bouts of walking and stair climbing into their daily lives not only burned as many calories as those who devoted larger blocks of time to recreational sports or leisure activities but also had similar reductions in heart disease risk. Small steps (literally!) add up to big gains.

Get More Mileage Out of Every Step

People who start walking start to love walking. In 2003, walking once again topped the National Sporting Goods Association's ranking of most popular sports. The appeal of walking is not only its simplicity but also its versatility. Like a simple black dress or a quality suit, you can strip it down or spiff it up to fit the occasion. Here are some tips to burn more fat, bust more stress, make more muscle, and have more fun with every step.

Try trekking

Wildly popular in Europe, trekking, or Nordic walking—striding with special rubber-tipped walking poles—is catching on at spas across the United States as a way to combine the calorie burn of cardiovascular exercise with the body sculpting of strength training. As each arm swings back, the tip of the pole lands and creates resistance that you must push against to propel yourself forward. Instead of flexing each muscle a

Walking Tip

Want to pick up the pace? Think short strides. One of the most common walking mistakes that people make is lengthening their strides to walk faster. When you do this, your front foot actually acts like a brake, jarring your joints and ultimately slowing you down. Instead, take short, quick, heel-to-toe strides. Your feet will roll forward more easily, and you'll move at greater speed without the stress.

few times in the gym, you activate every muscle longer, which improves muscular endurance and scorches fat.

Because pole walking engages your upper body muscles, it burns many more calories than regular walking. When researchers from the University of Wisconsin had 32 men and women perform a treadmill walking test—once with poles and once without—they found that the volunteers burned 22 percent more calories during the pole walk. The result: You can burn about 500 calories an hour while strengthening your shoulders, triceps, chest, back, abs, glutes, thighs, and calves. Even better, the poles help propel you, so walking actually feels easier. If you have a bum knee or sore hips, the poles help absorb the impact and can be the difference between the sofa and the sidewalk.

Belt it out

Walking with hand weights helps build muscle and burn calories, but too much weight can strain your shoulders and elbows. To safely increase upper body effort, try a PowerBelt, a wraparound device with retractable pulley cords that provide resistance. Simply strap it around your waist, hold on to the handles, and walk naturally, pulling the cord as you swing your arms. Again, because your upper body is working, your heart pumps harder, you burn more calories, and make more metabolism-revving muscle. PowerBelts cost roughly $80 and are sold on the Internet or at fitness stores.

Integrate exercises

For a change of pace integrate your favorite strength-training moves into your walk (see "Strength at Any Age" on page 149). Get moving for 2 minutes, then do 20 seconds of push-ups against a tree. Walk another 2 minutes, then do 20 seconds of walking lunges. This mix-and-match training raises your heart rate and burns more calories.

Achieve active intimacy

Make your daily walk a bonding ritual with your spouse. A study found that adults who exercise with a partner are more likely to exercise regularly and much less likely to quit than those who go it alone. Partners achieve what researchers call active intimacy—they grow closer and get in shape!

Meditate while you move

Meditating, or quieting your mind, is a proven heart-healthy habit. Taking a mental retreat can be easier and more effective when done while walking. The exertion will burn off stress hormones, and the repetitive movement will keep your mind focused and away from distracting thoughts and worries.

Start by walking a familiar route so you won't be distracted by your surroundings. Concentrate on feeling each foot strike the ground and focus on breathing rhythmically with your footsteps. As thoughts come to mind, allow them to pass through. You can also use this time to recite short prayers or give thanks. By the end of the walk, you should feel recharged and regenerated.

Figuring Out Your Walking Needs

How much time should you spend walking each day? Here's some helpful arithmetic. We've already noted that completely sedentary people walk about 3,000 steps in a day. Assuming that this is your base level as well, here's how much *extra* walking you need to do each day—measured for different paces—to reach specific step targets.

PACE	EXTRA WALKING TIME NEEDED TO REACH:		
	5,000 steps	7,000 steps	10,000 steps
Slow (80 steps per minute)	25 minutes	50 minutes	87 minutes
Regular (100 steps per minute)	20 minutes	40 minutes	70 minutes
Quick (120 steps per minute)	17 minutes	33 minutes	58 minutes
Fast (140 steps per minute)	14 minutes	29 minutes	50 minutes

Important: Your goal should be to get a majority of these extra steps during everyday activities—shopping, commuting, running errands, and otherwise going to and fro during the day. If you spend an extra 45 minutes a day on your feet as part of your daily routine and take a brisk, 15-minute pleasure walk after dinner, you'll easily get to 10,000 steps!

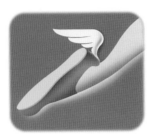

Picking Up the Pace

THE HARDEST PART of rolling a boulder down a hill is fighting the powerful forces of gravity and inertia to get it started. But once you give it a healthy heave-ho, it turns over, gains momentum, and becomes an almost unstoppable force.

Exercise is a lot like that: The toughest part is leaving the La-Z-Boy and getting in motion. Once you start moving, though, your energy goes up, your weight comes down, and you find yourself wanting to do even more—and when it comes to battling sitting disease and its ravaging effects, more is definitely better.

Although every little move you make helps nurture a healthier heart, you can build even more robust cardiovascular immunity by tossing vigorous activity, such as brisk walking, bicycling, and tennis, into the mix. When researchers from the Centers for Disease Control and Prevention analyzed data collected on 13,748 men and women ages 20 and older, they found that those who routinely got their tickers thumping hard three days a week were half as likely to have artery-damaging inflammation as those who did less vigorous activity.

If you already walk for exercise, picking up the pace can also help you get fit faster, according to a slew of scientific studies. In an eight-year analysis of 72,488 female nurses ranging in age from 40 to 65, researchers found that those who worked up a sweat for just 90 minutes a week—the equivalent of about 12 minutes a day—lowered their total heart disease risk by 30 to 40 percent. Similarly, the Harvard Health Professionals study of 44,452 men ages 40 to 79 found that those who ran for an hour or more each week dropped their heart disease risk by 42 percent. And researchers at the University of California, Berkeley, who studied 9,000 volunteers discovered that women who ran about 10 or more miles a week had slimmer waists and hips, lower blood pressure, and higher levels of good HDL cholesterol than those who exercised less intensely.

All Gain, No Pain

You don't have to (nor should you) heave and gasp and hurt to reap these rewards. New exercisers can raise their heart rates into the vigorous zone with little more than brisk walking. When University of Massachusetts researchers asked 84 overweight men and women to walk 1 mile at a pace that was "brisk but comfortable," the vast majority of the volunteers stepped right up to an

You don't have to heave and gasp and hurt to reap the rewards of exercise.

average 3.2 mph pace, which translates into hard to very hard intensity (70 to 100 percent of their maximum heart rates). The best part? "It was easier than people expected," says lead researcher Kyle McInnis, Sc.D. "They expected to have to suffer when really, they just had to go from a slow stroll to a brisk walk."

How do you know if you're working hard enough? Take the talk test. If you're able to recite the Pledge of Allegiance without hesitating, your exercise level is easy. If you can get it out phrase by phrase with little pauses for breath in between, you're right on target. If you can barely make it to "to the flag" without gasping for air, you're working too hard. You want to stay right in the middle.

Do You Need a Doctor's Okay?

Most people don't need to see a doctor before they start exercising, but for those with existing conditions, it's smart to get a medical okay before participating in energetic exercise. To find out if you need a checkup, review this checklist from the National Heart, Lung, and Blood Institute. If one or more of the statements apply to you, give your doctor a call before starting a new regimen.

- You have heart trouble or a heart murmur, or you have had a heart attack.

- You frequently have pain or pressure in the left or mid-chest area or the left neck, shoulder, or arm during or right after you exercise.

- You get breathless after only mild exertion.

- Your blood pressure is high and/or isn't under control, or you don't know whether

your blood pressure is normal.

- You have bone or joint problems, such as arthritis.

- You are over age 60 and not used to vigorous exercise.

- Your father, mother, brother, or sister had a heart attack before age 50.

- You have a medical condition not mentioned here that may need special attention in an exercise program.

11 Ways to Turn It Up

Here are several small steps that can infuse heart-healthy intensity into your everyday work and play. If you're new to vigorous activity, start slow and easy—be sure you're comfortable with the walking and general movement advice in the earlier chapters before trying to do more. Then introduce small advances, easing up when you feel you need a break. If you have high blood pressure, avoid caffeinated beverages before vigorous activity, since caffeine further increases heart rate and blood pressure. Finally, be enthusiastic, but don't overdo it. You want to feel good enough tomorrow to do it again.

1. Sneak in surges

The next time you're out walking, and you're warmed up, pick up the pace for 1 to 2 minutes. Slow down to take a breather, then repeat. You'll not only burn more calories, you'll also condition your body to feel comfortable at a faster pace so you'll be able to move more briskly every time you walk.

2. Power clean

A grimy house is better than Gold's Gym. Spin your favorite CDs, grab the cleaning supplies, and don't break 'til the last dust speck is spoken for. Alternate between upstairs and downstairs chores (instead of one floor at a time) to take advantage of the stairs—your home's best calorie burner.

3. Step to it

Whenever you see a set of stairs, take them. If there's time, go back down and take them again. If flexibility and balance aren't an issue, take two steps at a time. It's an easy way to get a burst of exercise intensity every day.

4. Head for the hills

Walking or riding a bike uphill means working harder against gravity—an added challenge for your muscles, heart, and lungs. Tackle some inclines (start with gentle ones) once or twice a week. When walking uphill, lean forward slightly to engage your powerful glute muscles. Walking downhill can be harder on your knees, so slow your pace, keep your knees slightly bent, and take shorter steps.

5. Dance, dance, dance

Whether you fancy the Pennsylvania Polka or a tango for two, dancing burns 480 calories an hour, uses your muscles in new ways, and puts joy in your heart. Some cardiologists say their patients who dance are the healthiest of the bunch. Make a date to go out twice a month.

6. Make a splash

The next time you're at the pool or beach, put down the murder mystery and dive in. Water is 800 times denser than air, so it provides instant intensity—and keeps you cool while you work out. Wade into the water about chest deep and try these moves.

Side kicks. Bend your right knee and then, without lowering it, kick out to the side, leaning toward the left as you kick. Lower your leg and repeat. Do 15 to 25 reps, then switch legs.

High steps. March quickly across the pool, raising your knees as high as possible as you step. Then march back.

Zigzag run. Pump your arms and legs and jog gently or run in a zigzag pattern across the pool and back. For the best results, keep your chest high and try not to bend forward.

7. Try some child's play

Kids are natural stop-and-go exercisers as they run, run, run, stop to catch a breath, and run some more. Play Frisbee, go swinging, or toss some horseshoes. You'll raise your heart rate and build priceless family bonds.

8. Find fast friends

Plan a few walks a week with someone who's just a hair fitter and faster than you. (That means you'll walk briskly enough to have a simple conversation, but not much more.) You'll push beyond your comfort zone and get fitter, faster yourself. Bonus: Exercising with a friend makes time fly, and you're more likely to stick to your routine if you make a date to do it with someone else.

9. Preprogram it

If you use a treadmill or other aerobic exercise equipment, choose the "interval" program to automatically add inclines, increased resistance, and higher-speed bursts to your workout.

10. Seek tougher terrain

Hiking trails, soft sand, and grassy fields all make you use more muscles and burn more calories than you would going at the same pace on asphalt. They're often in prettier places, too—so get off the beaten path whenever possible.

11. Get in the game

Resolve to take up one active hobby this year. Sporting hobbies such as tennis, cycling, and even golf (without the cart) include short bursts of heart-pumping effort. And they're fun, so time really flies. Here are some examples.

ACTIVITY	CALORIES BURNED PER HOUR*	SPECIAL BENEFITS
Bicycling	544	You feel like a kid again
Cross-country skiing	510	No winter weight gain
Gardening	340	Fresh, healthy veggies
Golfing (walking w/clubs)	374	Social contact; improves flexibility
Hiking	408	A chance to commune with nature
Ice skating/roller skating	408	Great family fun
Kayaking/canoeing	340	Builds upper body strength
Racquetball	476	You can play rain or shine
Scuba diving	476	Scenic and serene
Snowshoeing	544	Easy for all ages
Swimming	544	Low-impact; eases joint pain
Tennis	476	Builds bones
Volleyball (casual)	204	Improves eye-hand coordination

Based on a 150-pound person. Lighter people burn less; heavier people burn more.

Measuring Your Exertion

In the last chapter, we urged you to count your walking steps per day to track your level of activity. For those who are a little more serious about their exercise levels, there's a different measurement that we and nearly every fitness expert recommend you use: the amount of time you spend with your heart beating at an accelerated rate.

Here's the basic concept: Each of us has a maximum heart rate, above which we are overexerting the heart and putting ourselves at jeopardy. For most of us, maximum heart rate is the number 220 minus our age. So, if you are 60, your maximum heart rate is 160 beats per minute. With us so far?

Doctors and fitness experts recommend that while exercising, people reach and maintain roughly 60 to 65 percent of their maximum heart rates. For vigorous exercise, getting up to 80 percent of max is okay, but only if you are in great shape. The recommended quantity of exercise for healthy living? Keeping your heart rate at 60 percent of your max for at least 30 minutes a day. For our 60-year-old, that would be 96 beats per minute. In comparison, the average American has a resting heart rate of about 70 beats per minute.

Now, how can you possibly measure this? It's simple— with a heart-rate monitor. Like pedometers, heart-rate monitors are becoming ubiquitous in fitness circles. They run from $25 to $200, depending on the features, brand, and style, but all are wonderfully easy to use. First, you put a strap around your chest directly against your skin (once you put your shirt on, nobody can see it!). Next, you put a monitor on your wrist. Most look identical to wristwatches, and in fact, many include clocks; you can actually wear them all the time. But the monitor also receives signals from the chest strap, telling you your heart rate.

Most monitors are programmable. The most popular tool is the ability to program the target heart range you want to be in while exercising (say, 65 to 75 percent of max). The monitor then beeps if you exceed 75 percent or fall below 65 percent.

Do you need a heart-rate monitor? Not really. If you maintain the "breathing-hard-but-still-able-to-have-a-conversation" exertion level, you are almost certainly in the target range of 60 to 70 percent of max heart rate. If you're motivated by numbers or are getting serious about your workouts, though, by all means buy a monitor.

A heart-rate monitor is very easy to use and can help you be sure that you're getting the most out of your workout.

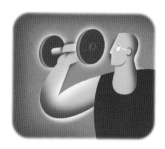

Strength at Any Age

WHEN HE TURNED 90, Jack LaLanne could still swim 10 miles at a time and crank out dozens of push-ups. His secret to seemingly endless vitality: Strength training. "As long as you have strong muscles, you're never old," decrees the godfather of fitness. Well, no muscle is more important than your heart, and strength training is as good for it as it is for your biceps.

Don't feel bad if this is the first time you're hearing that strength training helps your heart. Until recently, the only type of exercise that the medical community recognized as good for cardiovascular conditioning was endurance exercise such as walking, jogging, cycling, and swimming, which raise your heart rate and keep it elevated for an extended period of time. Today, every corner gym touts aerobic classes, such

as cardio kickboxing, to pull in the health-conscious crowd.

Well, new research shows that they may want to put "Heart-Pumping Iron" and "Artery-Clearing Arm Curls" on their marquees as well. Strength training not only helps muscle out the ill effects of sitting disease, it's also a simple step that wipes out nearly every heart attacker.

Strong-Arming Heart Disease

As anyone who's ever helped a friend move furniture or haul boxes of books knows, lifting weight makes your heart work harder, so the point that challenging your muscles also strengthens your heart is pretty obvious. But that's just the beginning of the benefits of strengthening your muscles. Research from the past five years shows that regular weight training can fend off at least four of the major heart attackers by improving triglyceride counts, cholesterol levels, blood pressure, and glucose metabolism and reducing body fat. In a landmark study of 44,000 men, Harvard researchers found that those who lifted weights for 30 minutes or more a week slashed their risk of heart disease by 23 percent.

How does the simple act of hoisting dumbbells deliver all these rewards? Here's what we now know.

✔ STRENGTH TRAINING STOPS METABOLISM MELTDOWN

A startling fact: Unless you take steps to stoke your metabolism—your body's calorie-burning ability—you can lose *a third to half* of your lean body mass and replace it with twice as much body fat by the time you're 65. That's a double whammy for heart health, since muscle tissue helps you burn off blood sugar, while excess fat raises your heart disease risk.

Like taking water from a swimming pool one bucket at a time, this muscle mass exodus happens so gradually that it often goes practically unnoticed for decades. It starts sometime around your 35th birthday, when levels of human growth hormone begin to fall. At the same time, family and work demands increase, leaving you with less time for physical fun than in decades past. This combination conspires to steal muscle tissue at the rate of about ½ pound a year. That may not sound like much, but consider this: Each day, muscle tissue burns about 15 times as many calories as fat does, even when you're not exercising. As muscle diminishes, so does your metabolism. The result: You gain fat.

Muscle Making 101

All this talk of sets and reps can sound intimidating to someone who's never routinely lifted anything heavier than a sack of flour, but it's really simple. Here's a primer to get you started.

Repetitions (reps). This term refers to the number of times you lift a weight or perform an exercise. Squatting up and down once is considered 1 repetition. Squatting 10 times is 10 reps.

Sets. This is the number of times you perform groups of reps. When we tell you to do 2 sets of 10 to 12 reps, we mean that you should do 10 to 12 consecutive reps, take a 30-second break, and do a second set of 10 to 12 reps.

Weight selection. As a general rule, the weight you lift should be heavy enough to make the final 2 or 3 repetitions feel tough. If you can do 15 reps without blinking an eye, pick a heavier weight. If you struggle to squeak out 6, go lighter. If an exercise is new to you, practice the movements without weights before your first workout.

Speed. Take your time. Each rep should take about 6 seconds, so slowly count 1-2-3 as you lift, pause a moment, and count 1-2-3 as you lower. By doing this, you'll be sure to use your muscles, not momentum, to do the work, and you'll get better results from your efforts.

Breathing. It may sound silly to remind someone to do something so automatic, but many people hold their breath while they lift—a risky practice if you have high blood pressure. For the best results, exhale as you push the weight against gravity and inhale as you move with gravity.

"Strength training is the best long-term method for increasing resting energy expenditure," says metabolism researcher Gary Hunter, Ph.D., of the University of Alabama at Birmingham. If you work every major muscle group twice a week, you can replace 5 to 10 years' worth of lost muscle in just a few months. In a study of 15 sedentary older adults, Dr. Hunter and his colleagues asked the volunteers to perform two sets of 10 to 12 strength-training exercises three days a week for six months. By the study's end, they boosted their metabolism by 7 percent, or 88 calories a day—enough to burn off more than 9 excess pounds in a year. And understand: That was without doing anything else. In other words, they lost weight independently of what they did or ate, solely because they had more muscle on their bodies (and the daily calorie figure doesn't include the calories burned while doing the exercise).

In a related study, Dr. Hunter found that women who followed a strength-training program for six months lost significant amounts of belly fat—the dangerous kind that elevates your odds of getting heart disease and diabetes.

✔ STRENGTH TRAINING IMPROVES CARDIOVASCULAR FITNESS

When your muscles get stronger, they can perform better with less oxygen. That means your heart doesn't have to race like Secretariat when you're doing everyday activities such as running up a flight of stairs or chasing tennis balls on the court. When a group of 46 adults lifted weights three times a week for six months, they not only got a lot stronger, they also improved their

Time Investment

Two sets of two strength-training exercises will take about 5 to 6 minutes to complete. Try doing your exercises while you watch your favorite prime-time program. (Keep your weights in a visible and accessible spot in the TV room as a gentle reminder.) That way you've invested zero extra time for a lifetime of heart benefits.

performance on a treadmill fitness test by about 25 percent. This University of Florida study was the first to show that strength training performs double duty by building aerobic fitness as well as strength.

✔ STRENGTH TRAINING FIGHTS FREE RADICALS

Lifting weights enhances your body's natural defense system against free radicals—natural by-products of metabolism that have been linked to chronic illnesses such as heart disease. In a study of free radical damage, researchers at the University of Florida had 62 men and women lift weights three times a week for six months. When they were given an exercise stress test at the end of the study, the weightlifters showed no evidence of damage from these molecular marauders, compared with a 13 percent increase in dangerous free radical activity among a similar group of adults who didn't lift weights.

✔ STRENGTH TRAINING BUILDS HEART POWER

Strength training conditions your heart to work better when you have to lift and carry heavy objects, so your blood pressure and heart rate are lower during everyday chores. What's more, strong muscles help share the load, so there's less demand on your heart when you carry groceries, shovel dirt, or clean the gutters.

Two a Day

In recognition of this growing list of strength-training benefits, the American Heart Association (AHA) now recommends that every American adult strength train all their major muscle groups about twice a week—yet barely 16 percent of Americans lift weights regularly. Surveys show that the biggest excuses are boredom and lack of time.

It's true, lifting weights isn't as exhilarating as cross-country skiing, and for many, it isn't nearly as interesting as watching a good episode of *Law & Order* or *The Sopranos*. But you needn't grind out hours in a dreary weight room to reap the rewards. With a few pieces of inexpensive equipment, you can build strong muscles and a healthy heart in as little as 5 minutes

Get On the Ball

Stability balls are excellent, versatile training tools. When you perform strength-training exercises on one of these inflated exercise balls, all your muscles, especially those in your core, kick in to help you maintain form and balance, so you get more benefit from each move. Plus, they sharpen your balance and coordination—something we all need as we get older. That said, the balls can seem somewhat odd and unstable for even seasoned exercisers at first. The following tips will help you start with confidence.

Buy the right size. Using a ball that's too big or too small will make these moves more difficult, or even dangerous if the ball is much too large. As a rule of thumb, when you sit on the top of the ball, your legs should be bent at 90 degrees when your feet are flat on the floor. Most balls include size charts on their packages. If you're 4 feet 8 inches tall or shorter, get a 45-centimeter ball; 4 feet 8 inches to 5 feet 3 inches, go with 55 centimeters; 5 feet 3 inches to 6 feet, buy a 65-centimeter ball; and taller than 6 feet, get a 75-centimeter ball.

Have a seat. Practice getting comfortable on the ball by simply sitting on it. Place it near a wall, put your hand on the wall for support, and have a seat. For better balance, place your feet wide apart for a more stable foundation. As you find your center of gravity and feel more stable, take your hand off the wall and practice sitting while raising your arms to the sides, then overhead.

Cheat a little. If balance is a problem when you start out, simply prop the ball against a wall and sit on it with your back to the wall. It will be less able to roll around beneath you while you build your balance and confidence.

Keep it properly inflated. The ball is hard to use if it's too squishy. It should be firm enough that it doesn't easily squeeze between your hands but soft enough that it gives a few inches when you sit on it.

Important note: Stability balls are designed to hold hundreds of pounds of pressure without popping, so use only these specially designed exercise balls. Don't substitute beach balls, department store children's toys, or other non-exercise-specific balls for these moves.

a day without ever leaving your living room. Heck, you don't even have to put on shoes or get out of your pajamas!

Spread out your routine so you perform two quick exercises a day. As you'll see in the following program, you still work all your major muscle groups twice a week, as recommended by the AHA, but the daily time commitment is minimal.

Consider this an important part of your 30-Minutes-A-Day commitment: Five minutes each morning or evening to do strength exercises. To get you going, we've created the Healthy Heart Strength Plan, one week's worth of exercises for your whole body. It's easy, it's fast, and it's proven to work!

What you'll need: Two sets of dumbbells, a lighter set for arm exercises and a heavier one for leg exercises. As a rule of thumb, women should use weights in the 5- to 15-pound range, and men should use 15- to 25-pound weights. You'll also need a stability ball, a large, inflated exercise ball that costs about $25. These balls are the best thing to happen to strength training since forged steel. You can not only use a stability ball as a substitute for a weight bench, you can also do dozens of exercises using just it and your body weight to strengthen and tone every major muscle, especially your "core"—the abdomen, back, and hips. Both dumbbells and stability balls can be purchased at any major sporting goods store, or you can comparison shop online at www.balldynamics.com, where you'll find numerous brands. (For more on using a stability ball, see "Get On the Ball" on page 152.)

What to do: Follow the program starting on page 154, performing two sets of 10 to 12 repetitions of each exercise. Rest for 30 seconds between sets. New to strength training? See "Muscle Making 101" on page 150 for more advice on getting started.

Bonus: You'll find that these moves become easier in a month or two as your body adapts to the workload. Studies show that strength training is most effective when you "surprise" your muscles with new challenges every 8 to 12 weeks.

> You can build strong muscles and a healthy heart in as little as 5 minutes a day without leaving your living room.

Monday

Back and Biceps

Your back is made up of multiple layers of muscles that help you lift and pull as well as hold your body upright. Your biceps are the muscles in the fronts of your upper arms that you use to hoist shopping bags and small children. These exercises target those two muscle groups.

CURL AND PRESS

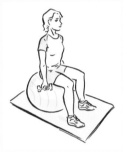 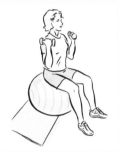 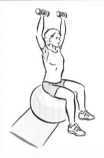

SIT ON the stability ball or a chair with your feet flat on the floor about shoulder-width apart. Hold a dumbbell in each hand with your arms at your sides, palms facing out.

KEEPING your upper body stable, bend your elbows and curl weights toward your shoulders.

IMMEDIATELY TURN your wrists so your palms face out in front of you and press the weights straight overhead. Pause, then

slowly reverse the move, lowering the weights to your shoulders, rotating your palms, and lowering the weights to your sides.

KEEP your shoulders down as you curl and lift; don't let them hunch up toward your ears

BACK FLY

SIT ON the edge of the stability ball or a chair with your feet together and flat on the floor.

HOLD a dumbbell in each hand. Keeping your back flat, bend forward at the waist and lower your chest to about 3 or 4 inches above your knees, letting your arms hang down on either side of your legs with your hands by your feet.

SQUEEZE your shoulder blades and raise the weights out to the

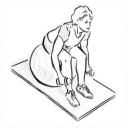 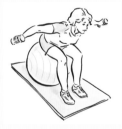

sides until your arms are outstretched parallel to the floor.

Pause, then slowly return to the starting position.

Tuesday

Chest and Triceps

Your chest is composed of fan-shaped muscles that span from shoulders to sternum and help you push carts and hug loved ones. Your triceps are also "pushing" muscles located on the backs of your upper arms—notoriously weak and saggy spots.

STABILITY BALL PUSH-UPS

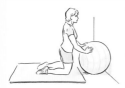 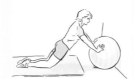 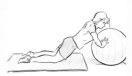

PLACE the stability ball against a wall, then kneel in front of it so it's between you and the wall.

PLACE your hands on the ball so they're directly below your shoulders. Walk back on your knees

until your body forms a straight line from your head to your knees. You should be leaning forward into the ball.

KEEPING your torso straight and your abs contracted (concentrate

on pulling your belly button to your spine), bend your elbows and lower your chest toward the ball.

STOP when your elbows are in line with your shoulders. Pause, then return to the starting position.

CHAIR DIPS

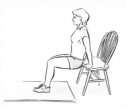 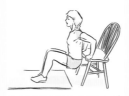 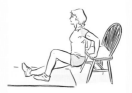

PROP a sturdy chair against a wall and sit with the heels of your hands on the edge of the seat. Inch your buttocks off the seat, supporting your weight with your hands.

KEEPING your shoulders down and your back straight, bend your elbows back and dip your body toward the floor as far as comfortably possible (even if it's just a few inches). Push back up to the starting position.

TO MAKE the move more challenging, extend one leg and plant the heel of that foot on the floor in front of you.

Friday
Chest and Triceps

Back to the muscles exercised Tuesday, with some fresh strengthening moves.

CHEST FLY

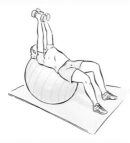 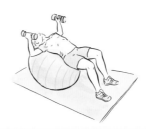

LIE BACK on the stability ball so it supports your torso from your neck to your midback, with your knees bent and your feet flat on the floor. Hold the dumbbells over your chest with your arms extended and your palms facing each other. Keep your elbows slightly bent.

SLOWLY OPEN your arms to the sides, lowering the weights until your upper arms are parallel to the floor. Pause, then slowly return to the starting position. Keep your shoulders down and back throughout the move.

TRICEPS PRESSBACK

SIT ON the stability ball with your knees bent and your feet flat on the floor. Hold the dumbbells in front of you with your arms bent at 90-degree angles and your elbows at your sides. Keeping your back straight, bend slightly from the hips.

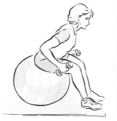 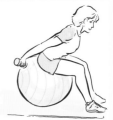

STRAIGHTEN your arms and extend the weights behind your back, turning your palms toward the ceiling once your arms are fully extended. Pause, then return to the starting position.

Saturday
Legs and Core

A return to the muscles exercised on Wednesday, but with interesting variations.

STABILITY BALL LEG CURLS

SIDE PLANK

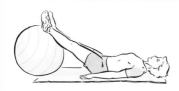

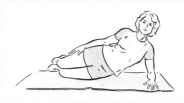

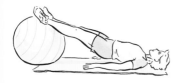

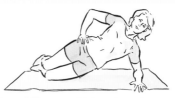

LIE ON your left side with your knees bent. Bend your left arm so your forearm is extended in front of you perpendicular to your body, then lift your torso off the floor. Your upper body should form a straight line from your hips to your shoulders.

PLACE your right hand on your hip and hold for 5 to 15 seconds. Return to the starting position, then repeat on other side. Work up to holding on each side for 30 to 60 seconds. Perform just one rep per set.

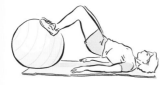

LIE ON your back on the floor, extend your legs, and place your heels on top of the stability ball. Rest your arms on the floor by your sides, palms down.

PRESS your heels into the ball and lift your buttocks a few inches off the floor.

BEND your knees, using your heels to pull the ball toward your buttocks so your feet end up flat on the ball. Pause, then return to the starting position.

**Sunday:
Rest Day!**
Kick back and give yourself a pat on the back.

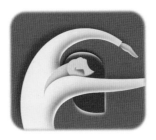

The Restorative Power of Stretching

AS TODDLERS, most of us were so flex-ible that we could easily touch our chins with our big toes.

As adults, many of us are so stiff that it hurts our joints merely to clip our toenails.

What causes us to lose so much flexi-bility over time? Easy: Sitting disease.

The fact is, the average sedentary person will lose a quarter to a third of his range of motion during his adult life—a change that can dramatically curtail activity levels and contribute to a weakened heart. Because flexibility creeps away slowly over the years, we barely notice its departure until we sud-denly realize we can tie our shoes only if we are sitting.

This is one of the amazing things about the human body: The more we use our mus-cles and joints, the longer they last. We're not like machines, which wear out with use.

When we're active, our muscles, bones, and joints get stronger, repair themselves, and adapt, but when we live sedentary lives, our moving parts slowly lose these abilities.

"If your life revolves around sitting on a sofa, sitting in a car, and sitting at a desk all day, you can easily lose 75 percent of your normal range of motion by the time you're 60," says physical therapist Vincent Perez, director of sports therapy at Columbia-Pres-byterian Eastside in New York City. "Then it's a vicious cycle. It's hard to move, so you don't try, and you become stiffer and more sedentary. The less active your daily life is, the more important it is to stretch."

Aside from making your muscles more limber so you can enjoy a more active life, stretching also helps tame high blood pres-sure and insulin resistance by lowering stress. Your muscles are equipped with stretch receptors that are in constant communication with your brain about your overall level of tension. When your muscles are chronically tight, your brain gets the message that you're under constant stress. Stretching promotes muscle relaxation, which in turn sends an "A-OK" to the brain, signaling that all is well.

Open Your Muscles

One look in the mirror will tell you that the body's tissues change as we age. Just as our skin thins and gets drier with time, so do our muscles and connective tissues. With less fluid keeping them plump and supple, muscles lose their elasticity and grow shorter and tighter. Short, rigid muscles act like tourniquets, constricting circulation so blood vessels can't deliver nutrients and carry out waste as well as they should. As waste builds up, calcifications (hard knots) form, which leave us feeling as stiff as the Tin Man after a rainy day.

The result is that we literally get stuck in the hunched-over positions most Americans assume for hours each day as we read, type, drive, eat, cook, and clean. "Poor posture is rampant, and the main culprit is inflexibility," says Perez. "Many people dismiss bad posture as just an aesthetic problem, but hunching and slumping do more than look bad. They cause a whole series of problems, like muscle imbalances, headaches, back pain, and disk degeneration." Poor posture even affects your breathing, making it shallower than it should be because your lungs can't fully expand when your chest is collapsed forward. Hunching forward tends to cause people to feel physically and emotionally bad.

(continued on page 164)

Stay Active Without Injury

Arrive early at a soccer match or football game, and you will see the athletes twisting, bending, reaching for the sky, and dropping toward their toes. For active people, stretching has long been the hallmark of injury prevention. Recent studies, however, have cast a wide shadow of doubt on that conventional wisdom. Just last year, the Centers for Disease Control and Prevention (CDC) declared that stretching before exercise provides no protection against sports injuries.

Before you terminate your toe touches, though, take note: The CDC was referring to acute injuries—sprains, pulls, and strains—not painful chronic conditions, such as Achilles tendinitis, that can arise from having chronically tight muscles and connective tissue. Stretching is still essential for general flexibility and can help you avoid long-term aches and pains. It can also improve your performance. When you regularly stretch your muscles, you increase your range of motion, which allows you to produce more power and makes you more balanced and agile when you work and play.

Finally, studies show that stretching after exercise is like wringing the lactic acid and accumulated metabolic waste out of your muscles. The result: Less post-exercise muscle soreness, so you'll feel ready to go the next day. The stretches in this chapter will help keep you walking, biking, and playing tennis without pain.

4 Minutes to Flexibility

Stretching is a lot like flossing: Everyone agrees it's a good idea, but few people actually take the time or make the effort to do it. The American Council on Exercise recently named neglecting to stretch the number one mistake that active folks make.

Here's your chance to make amends with your neglected muscles. The following is a stretching sequence you can do practically anywhere in just 4 minutes. Although you can do these moves at any time of day, we suggest doing them after your morning shower. Like taffy, your muscles are most "stretchy" when they're nice and warm. Perform the sequence twice, flowing from move to move and holding each stretch for 15 seconds. Stretch only until you feel a slight "pull" or stretch in the muscle; you should feel tension relief, never pain. When you're finished, you'll be loose, limber, and relaxed to start the day

SKY REACH

Muscles and joints stretched: Back, shoulders, sides (obliques), abs, and hands.

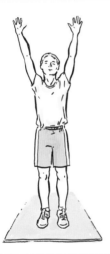

STAND straight with your feet about hip-width apart. Extend your arms overhead so your fingers point straight at the ceiling. Rise on the balls of your feet and spread your fingers, stretching upward to make your body as long and tall as possible. Tilt your chin slightly to look at the ceiling. Hold, then return to the starting position.

WALL STRETCH

Muscles and joints stretched: Calves, hamstrings, back, and shoulders.

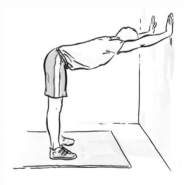

STAND a few feet away from a wall and place your hands on it, shoulder-width apart. Move your feet back until you're leaning into the wall and you feel a gentle stretch in your calves. Slowly press your hips back and press your heels into the floor so you feel a stretch in your back as well as your calves. Hold, then return to the starting position.

Muscles and joints stretched: Chest, arms, and wrists.

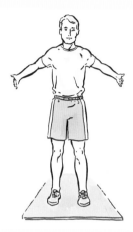

STAND with your feet shoulder-width apart and your knees slightly bent for support. Keep your back straight and your chin level. Slowly extend your arms up and to the sides until they're just below shoulder level. With your palms facing forward, gently stretch your arms behind you. When you've pulled back as far as comfortably possible, bend your wrists back until you feel a stretch in the fronts of your upper arms. Hold, then slowly return to the starting position.

Muscles and joints stretched: Sides (obliques), inner thighs, hamstrings, and neck.

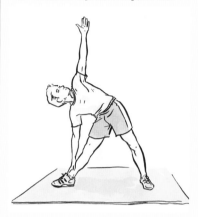

STAND with your feet wider than shoulder-width apart and point your left foot forward and your right foot to the side. Extend your arms straight out to the sides at shoulder level, then bend to the right, reaching for your right shin with your right hand. Extend your hand as far down your leg as comfortably possible while reaching toward the ceiling with your left hand. Turn your head slightly to look at the ceiling. Hold, then return to the starting position and repeat, stretching to the opposite side.

Muscles and joints stretched: Hips, buttocks, and thighs.

STAND straight and place your hands on a chair back or tabletop for support. Raise your right leg and place your right ankle on your lower left thigh, right above the knee. Bend your left leg, move back slightly as if starting to sit, and gently press your right knee toward the floor, feeling the stretch in your right hip and the back of your thigh. Hold, then return to the starting position and repeat on the other side.

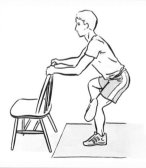

When you progressively stretch your muscles through their full range of motion, you open the channels, promote circulation, and encourage efficient nutrient transport and swift waste removal from those tissues. Stretching will also increase the synovial fluid (the body's natural oil that lubricates your joints) in your hinges and sockets, which helps keep your joints healthy and moving smoothly. When your muscles, tendons, and ligaments are supple, your posture improves, and everything from picking socks off the floor to driving golf balls feels more effortless.

No matter how long you've been stationary, stretching can help restore your mobility. In a small study at the University of California, Davis, researchers found that men and women who practiced yoga twice a week broke free of the Quasimodo hunch and improved their spinal flexibility—the ability to arch backward—by an astonishing 188 percent. But you don't have to spend hours twisting into pretzel-like positions. Even a few minutes of simple stretches a day can restore lost flexibility by 10 to 15 percent, says Perez.

The Perpetual Stretch

Routines such as the one given here are terrific in that they target all the major muscle groups and give you maximum benefit in little time. But stretching is the type of activity that is good anytime, anywhere. It gives you a boost out of the afternoon doldrums. It brings blood to your hands and wrists when you've been typing or cooking a

Are You Limber?

People in their fifties shouldn't be expected to bend like pretzels, but neither should they be as stiff as pretzel sticks. Here are reasonable estimates of how limber you should be, given a healthy, moderately active lifestyle.

- You should be able to sit on the edge of a chair (one leg extended, one bent) and bend over to tie the shoe on the foot of the extended leg.
- You should be able to scratch a mosquito bite between your shoulder blades by reaching either behind your head or up from your waist.
- You should be able to remove a snug T-shirt by crossing your arms in front of your body, grasping the bottom hem, and pulling the shirt off in a smooth overhead motion.
- You should be able to turn your head and look directly over either shoulder.
- You should be able to reach behind you far enough with both arms to slip into a coat someone is holding behind you.

little too long. It prepares you for walks, lifts your spirits, and gets you on your feet (yet one more way to battle sitting disease). Thus, while we recommend that you follow our 4-minute routine, we also advocate stretching all through your day and evening, too. Check out some yoga-based stretches in magazines and books. Just be sure to stretch safely and gently and to hold each position for at least 15 seconds if you want your muscles and joints to benefit.

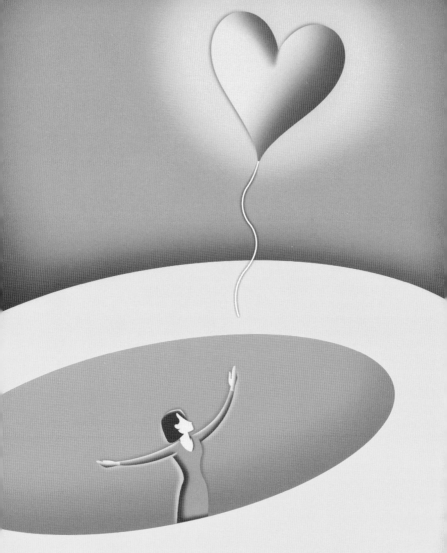

5 Nurturing a
Happy Heart

The evidence is conclusive: Your emotions and attitudes have a direct influence on the health of your heart. Consider it another reason to enjoy life more.

How to
Be Kind
to Your
Heart

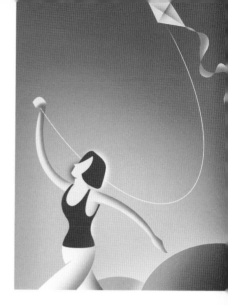

IMAGINE THAT YOU had a cherished pet. You would probably care for her in every way imaginable. You'd feed her healthy, nutritious food in appropriate portions; give her plenty of exercise; and provide her with a warm, comfortable place to sleep. But those are just the basic necessities. Like most doting pet owners, you'd also shower her with affection, play games with her, soothe her during stressful times, and provide lots of happiness and fun in the interest of a long, healthy life.

Shouldn't you treat your heart as well as you'd treat a pet? The analogy is less of a stretch than you might think. As with a dog or cat, whether your heart thrives or falls ill largely depends on your care, love, nurturing, and kindness.

In the long run, being kind to your heart is better than any medicine money can buy.

In the groundbreaking Lifestyle Heart Trial, researchers from California Pacific Medical Center followed nearly 50 men and women with moderate to severe coronary disease for five years. Half of the group did not take medications but rather made lifestyle changes that included healthy eating, exercise, stress management, support meetings, and quitting smoking. The other half followed the usual medical regimen that focused on medication and more subtle lifestyle changes. At the study's end, the lifestyle group's arteries were actually about 8 percent clearer, while the usual-care group's clogging had worsened by almost 28 percent despite medication. What's more, the volunteers in the usual-care group experienced twice as many cardiac events, such as arrhythmias or heart attacks, as those who turned to healthier lifestyles.

6 Steps to a Happy Heart

It's interesting how many people shun this type of emotional-health advice. Heart health requires more serious steps, they say. Medicine, supplements, rigorous diets, formal exercise regimens—that's how you guarantee health, according to the doctors. Well, don't fall into that trap. Research strongly confirms the healing power of a good attitude, a good laugh, a good round of prayer. This is not "alternative medicine" or the wishful thinking of youth-seeking baby boomers. The finest universities and researchers have spoken: For a healthy heart, happiness does matter. Consider the following six steps essential to the 30-Minutes-A-Day Plan.

1. Believe

Faith, whether in a higher being, the power of nature, or even yourself, is both grounding and healthy. A big part of this is optimism. People who use words such as *joy* and *hope* to describe their attitudes toward life outlive their more pessimistic counterparts by a decade. No matter what your situation, the power to put down anger and embrace the good things in life lies in your hands.

2. Enjoy life

Sometime between leaving our parents' homes and signing off on a 30-year mortgage on our own, we stop having as much fun as we used to. We all have serious adult responsibilities, but we also have the responsibility to our heart to let loose and have some childlike fun. Studies show that people whose lives are filled with laughter are much less likely to have heart disease.

3. Practice relaxing rituals

As life gets more hurried, stress rises, and heart disease follows. You can't change the world, but you can change your response to it. Daily rituals such as meditation, yoga, visualization, quiet time, bedtime relaxation, and even just walking a dog can quell stress and reduce your risk of heart disease.

4. Indulge moderately

Those who savor a glass of wine with dinner now and again may lower their heart disease risk by up to 40 percent, generally enjoying a higher quality of life than both those who abstain completely and those who don't know when to say when.

5. Create a safe haven

They say that home is where the heart is. Well, make yours a refuge for your hardworking ticker. Set up soothing surroundings with flowers, plants, good music, a sleep-inducing bedroom, and some quiet space where you can escape when you need to collect your thoughts. Spending most of your time relaxed instead of stressed can slice your heart disease risk in half.

6. Share yourself

Hearts are happiest when they're in the company of others. Make time for family and friends and get involved with the community through volunteer work, religious services, and/or charitable contributions. Your heart will thank you.

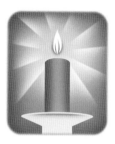

Faith

WANT TO ADD SEVEN years to your life? Bow your head and say a prayer. Over the years, scientists around the globe have conducted more than 1,200 studies, all of which point to a positive relationship between spirituality and longevity. Nurturing your spiritual health through prayer, faith, and religious involvement has been associated with a seven-year increase in longevity—a life span benefit equivalent to that of not smoking cigarettes!

Although the medical community has historically turned a skeptical eye to the power of prayer, scientists are increasingly recognizing the biological benefits of belief. Studies show that attending worship services slows heart rate, alleviates stress, and promotes general wellness. Research from Duke, Dartmouth, and Yale universities shows a strong connection between heart

health and religious activity. In one study, people undergoing open-heart surgery who reported feeling strength and comfort from their religion were three times more likely to survive than those who had no such spiritual grounding. Another study reported that heart patients were 14 times more likely to die following surgery if they didn't have a spiritual connection.

Of course, it would be unrealistic to suggest that you "find religion" to save your heart. Even if you're not interested in formal religious services, though, nurturing your spiritual side through activities such as community involvement, prayer, communing with nature, and meditation has clear benefits. People who tend to their inner selves are less likely to drink excessively, smoke, or lead socially isolated lives. Even skeptics acknowledge that at the very least, there's probably a powerful placebo effect connected to faith. That is, people may get better simply because they believe they will.

The Power of Prayer

Praying for the sick or dying is a common practice among people of all faiths. Praying for yourself or knowing others are praying for you can help improve your ability to cope with and reduce your anxiety about whatever is ailing you. Some scientists also believe that prayer or positive thinking boosts immunity and improves the overall function of the cardiovascular, central nervous, and hormonal systems.

In a groundbreaking study of 150 men and women undergoing emergency angioplasty (a highly stressful invasive procedure), researchers at Duke found that those who were prayed for by others had the lowest rate—up to a 25 to 30 percent reduction—of adverse outcomes, such as death, heart failure, or heart attacks. Although a follow-up study failed to replicate these findings, faith researchers remain intrigued by the potential power of prayer.

Some scientists argue that we are hardwired for faith. Harvard scientist Herbert Benson, M.D., has studied prayer and meditation for 30 years. During that time, he has documented through MRI brain scans that prayer literally envelops the brain in what he calls quietude, a state in which the nervous system, heart rate, blood pressure, metabolism, and all basic body systems become relaxed. No matter whether you recite the Catholic rosary or a Buddhist meditation, the effect is the same.

Find Your Soulful Side

Whether you're Christian, Jewish, Muslim, Hindu, or just not sure, you can reap the rewards of some spiritual celebration. One obvious way is to attend religious services, but there are many other means of feeding your soul.

Meditate on the move. Research at the University of Massachusetts Medical Center showed that meditation eases anxiety and lowers blood pressure. It's also a tool used in most religions to bring you closer to a higher spiritual power. People mistakenly believe that you need to sit still to meditate, but meditating on the move can be just as effective, if not more so, because exercise sets the stage for increased calm by lowering stress hormones and bringing lots of fresh oxygen into your body. Take a few minutes during your daily walk to calm and clear your mind by focusing on your footsteps and the feeling and sound of your breath moving in and out of your lungs.

Help others. Helping a worthy cause, whether through financial contributions or volunteering your time, deepens your connection to humanity and promotes a feeling of greater purpose. If time permits, donate your services by delivering food to the needy, walking dogs at an animal shelter, or teaching someone to read. Or, once a month, gather up old blankets, coats, and surplus canned goods from your closets and cupboards and deliver them to a local shelter. Check the local or community section of your newspaper for listings of needed volunteer services. Other small but heartlifting ways to positively touch others include writing letters to old friends, teachers, or even politicians; doing random acts of kindness for others, be it opening doors for someone carrying grocery bags or giving up a parking space to a mom with several kids in her car; or offering frequent (but honest) praise to family, friends, and coworkers.

Take a walk in the woods. Few people can walk through a forest, hike up a mountain, bask in the ocean, or even sit by a flower garden without feeling the beauty and power of a larger force around them. Make it a point to get outside once a day, even if it's just to sit under a tree in your backyard. Don't limit yourself to daytime, either. A nighttime excursion offers different sounds, the night sky, and a sense of calm you just can't experience on a daylight walk.

Say it out loud. In an Italian study of men and women reciting either the Ave Maria or a yoga mantra, researchers found that both appeared to slow breathing rhythms to 6 breaths a minute (the average rate is about 16 to 20 breaths per minute) as well as synchronize breathing rate with cardiovascular rhythms—both of which calm the central nervous system and induce a feeling of well-being. Interestingly, these effects weren't present when the mantra and prayer were not recited aloud. If you use meditative phrases, speaking them may increase their effect.

Give thanks. Once a day, whether first thing in the morning, before dinner, or at bedtime, take a moment to give thanks for everything you appreciate in your life. Actively expressing appreciation for essentials such as food and your family, home, and job can remind you of what's really important and how fortunate you are while

Stock Your Spiritual Pantry

Since the beginning of time, places of worship have used music, incense, and candles to help set the spiritual stage. To help feed your soul at home, stock up on similar items that are known to heighten the devotional mood.

- **Candles:** Nothing soothes like a flickering flame.

- **CDs:** Whether gospel, country ballads, or violin concertos, music opens your heart, alters your brain waves, and connects you to your spiritual self.

- **Symbols or statues:** Crosses, Stars of David, Buddha figures, statues of saints, and other religious symbols are powerful reminders that you are not alone.

- **Flowers and/or plants:** Living things evoke the beauty and simplicity of the natural world.

- **Incense:** The rising smoke from burning incense historically symbolized prayers rising up to God; the scent is also soothing. If you don't like smoke, try steaming potpourri instead.

spiritually connecting you to the world at large. While you're giving thanks, take a moment to extend good wishes and send prayers or positive energy to others.

Express yourself. For many people, journaling—recording private thoughts and observations in a diary—is a way to stay in touch with their spiritual needs. Others feel inspired when they paint, practice photography, or even refinish furniture. Whatever medium you choose, expressing yourself artistically is a sure way to soothe your soul.

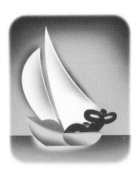

Enjoying Life

WHEN WAS THE LAST time you felt lighthearted—or were heartbroken? All of our heartfelt emotions—from love to loneliness, happiness to hate—affect not only the way we see the world but also how long we spend living in it.

In a 15-year study of 678 nuns living and teaching in Minnesota, researchers from the University of Kentucky found that those who most often used positive words such as *happy*, *joy*, *love*, *glad*, and *content* when describing their lives in letters and diaries lived as much as 10 years longer than those who expressed fewer positive emotions. The researchers concluded that good feelings can act as a biological shield against daily stresses that otherwise take their toll in the form of high blood pressure, heart disease, and more.

Happiness helps you live longer even if you already have heart disease. For 11 years, Duke University researchers tracked the emotions and overall health of 866 men and women (average age 60) who had undergone cardiac catheterization. Those who most frequently checked off positive descriptions such as "intense joy," "optimism," "lightheartedness," and "ability to laugh easily" on a questionnaire about their personalities and emotional states were 20 percent less likely to die of any cause, including heart disease, than those who picked less positive phrases.

Type A-nger

Just as all those happy feelings can act as powerful life extenders, negative emotions can have the opposite effect. Anger, impatience, and hostility significantly raise your risk of heart disease. In a large-scale Northwestern University study, researchers enrolled 3,308 men and women, ages 18 through 30, from different cities throughout the country and tracked their mental and physical well-being for 15 years. The participants who scored highest for feelings of impatience and/or hostility had an astonishing 84 percent greater risk of developing high blood pressure than those who scored lowest.

A similar seven-year study of 1,300 men found that those who reported the most intense levels of anger were three times more likely to have heart attacks and/or episodes of chest pain than those with the least anger. Other research has pinned strong feelings of hostility to a 30 percent increase in the likelihood of developing atrial fibrillation, a heart disorder that increases the risk of blood clots.

Why is hostility so hurtful? Think about what happens when you get really mad. Your face flushes. Your hands quiver. You clench up. Internally, the effects are equally profound. As you shake your fist at that idiot driver who cut you off, the arteries supplying blood to your heart constrict. Your blood becomes stickier and thus more likely to clot. Your blood sugar spikes. Surging adrenaline sends your heart rate soaring. Repeat this cycle over and over—with your darn boss, your inconsiderate neighbors, those noisy kids—and the physical wear and tear contributes to higher homocysteine

Our heartfelt emotions— from love to loneliness, happiness to hate—can affect how long we live.

levels, elevated cholesterol, high blood pressure, and ultimately, heart disease.

Likewise, spending each day in a haze of gloom and doom hurts your heart, too. In a long-term study of 1,200 men, researchers from Johns Hopkins University in Baltimore, Maryland, found that men who were depressed (see "Are You Depressed?" on page 175) were twice as likely as men without depression to develop coronary artery disease or have heart attacks 15 years later.

Choosing Happiness

Why are so many of us so sad and angry? There's no question that we're born with certain innate personality characteristics, but experts say that much of how we respond to the world around us is learned. Almost all of us face the same grim headlines, relentless mortgage payments, daily traffic jams, and never-ending bills in the mail. Some of us have decided that this is just what life is, and we skate through it with a shrug and a smile. Others choose to take such everyday affronts personally and get angry at the infinite injustices of modern-day life. Understand this simple truth: Which path you take is nothing more than a personal choice. Nothing compels you to be angry—except yourself.

We're not telling you to attempt a personality transformation as a way to protect your heart. We are who we are. Rather, we suggest that in those rare moments when you're confronted with a challenging situation, you pause before reacting in your usual way, consider your choices, and choose a more positive, life-affirming response. After all, isn't life better when you're smiling rather than frowning? It's easier than you think to walk away from anger.

To get you started, here are proven methods to increase everyday joy and, as a result, improve your heart's health.

Let it out. A nine-year study of 2,500 men showed that those who bottled up their anger were up to 75 percent more likely to develop coronary artery disease than those who vented their frustration. The next time you're hot under the collar, find a friend and let off some steam.

Take a 10-second time-out. That old advice to count to 10 may sound corny, but it has a sound biological basis. When you count, your brain activity shifts to the frontal cortex, the area of rational thought, and away from the emotionally charged limbic system, where there's little control over emotions. That's why you feel better able to cope after a 10 count. You can increase the effectiveness of this exercise by taking deep belly breaths, which trigger the relaxation response.

Evoke feelings of love. Studies at the Institute of HeartMath in California found that feelings of love actually make your heart beat more smoothly and regularly. Our suggestion: Do something each day to bring a sustained, loving smile to your face. Download a couple of great photos of your kids when they were toddlers to your computer and call them up when you need a break. Provide hugs galore to your spouse. Listen to some classic Sinatra love songs. Don't want to leave this to chance? Try something called the loving-kindness meditation, which you can do anywhere. Simply:

- Take a break from what you're doing and focus on your heart.

- Recall an experience during which you felt happiness, love, and appreciation.

- Breathe deeply and feel your heart lighten as you re-experience those feelings.

Such heartfelt meditation can even out your heart rhythm in just 60 seconds, according to HeartMath researchers.

Give the benefit of the doubt. The instant you feel rising anger at a salesclerk or restaurant server, for example, pause and reflect on the big picture. Are the store's crazy return policies really the clerk's fault? Is it reasonable to expect a high-schooler on a summer job at the grocery store to be an expert on each brand of ham at the deli counter? Does the government clerk have any power to break the rules as you'd like? Lashing out at people rarely results in getting what you want, and it's often unfair. Worst of all, it transfers your anger to a second person. Feeling empathy cools anger quickly (and amazingly, often gets better results!).

Drop the ball (at least one). Anger, frustration, and impatience peak when we try to do too many things at once. Examine your to-do list each day and eliminate the lowest-priority item. In doing so, you'll forge the habit of focusing on only what's most important, without sweating the small stuff.

Let go of one grudge. University of Wisconsin researchers found that men with coronary artery disease who had unresolved anger from childhood, war, domestic conflicts, or professional problems could improve blood flow to their hearts through forgiveness training. Staying steamed increases adrenaline levels while snuffing out the feel-good hormone serotonin. Forgiveness releases that bottled-up anger and creates a healthier hormone balance. Today, choose one incident you're still stewing about and decide to let it go. Experts emphasize that forgiveness doesn't mean excusing bad behavior or even reconciling with the offender. It means that you decide not to let that incident or person have control over your life or the power to hurt your heart. It may take time and maybe even outside assistance, but by deciding to forgive, you're halfway there.

Forgive yourself, too. No one can beat us up better than we do. While you're working on forgiving others, remember to go easy on yourself. You can't change the past, only improve the present, and that means giving yourself a break.

Have fun. When is the last time you had fun? If a recent memory doesn't pop into your mind, it's time to ink some fun into your calendar. It doesn't have to be elaborate, just something you look forward to. Once a week, set up a golf date, rent a funny movie, or take your kids or grandkids to the park. You'll feel less bogged down by daily life if you regularly reward yourself with good times.

Give and take control. We can't control world events, corporate downsizing, bad weather, and the ill-advised actions of others, yet many of us take such affronts personally. Learn to let them go without anger or guilt. Place things that are out of your control in the hands of a "higher power," whether that means God or simply fate (see "Faith" on page 169), then take control of what you can. You can't make offensive people be polite, for example, but you can choose to avoid them in the future.

Are You Depressed?

A majority of Americans are overweight, but a much smaller percentage fall into the category of being obese, a well-defined medical condition that needs to be treated by a doctor. Likewise, virtually all of us get the blues now and then, but depression is a serious medical condition that requires serious treatment. Left unchecked, depression sets up a vicious cycle of not exercising, increasing worries, weight gain, and fatigue that exacts a high toll on your heart. Heed these signs of depression.

- Being in a sad mood most days
- Loss of appetite
- Loss of energy
- Fatigue
- Problems sleeping or sleeping excessively
- Inability to concentrate or make decisions
- Feelings of worthlessness or guilt
- Weight loss or gain
- Lack of interest in pleasurable activities and/or sexual activity
- Thoughts of death or suicide

If you believe you may be depressed, see your doctor. Depression isn't merely a mental state; it's usually linked to chemical imbalances that can be corrected with medication and lifestyle adjustments.

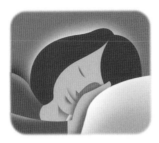

Defeating Stress

STRESS. THE WORD alone is enough to conjure up images of clammy palms, sweaty brows, and blood pressure pills—but in the right dose, stress can be good. Think about it. A violin string without stress is dull and lifeless, yielding no resonance or melody to the touch. If it's wound too tight, it snaps. With just the right amount of stress, the string sings, creating energetic, harmonious music.

That's how life is, too. A little bit of self-created tension generates the mental and physical energy you need to accomplish goals and meet dreams. If there's too much, however (and most of us are swimming in it), your heartstrings do their own "snapping." Research shows that unchecked stress leads to a cascade of symptoms, including insulin resistance; increased abdominal fat; elevated blood pressure; and "heart rate variability," a condition that hampers your heart's ability to react properly, upping your risk for sudden cardiac arrest.

Your goal: Make small changes in your lifestyle to maintain healthy tension while reducing excess stress so your life (and your heart) keeps humming along happily and productively.

Hurry Up and Worry

You're driving on a freeway and someone cuts you off, forcing you to slam on the brakes. Your passengers gasp, and your heartbeat surges. This type of event is called acute stress, referring to unexpected, one-time bursts of fear or excitement that trigger your body to tense up and prepare for a fight with or flight from danger.

Relax, drivers: An occasional episode of acute stress isn't what doctors are most concerned with. Rather, it's what's called chronic stress—worries and concerns that linger for days, months, or years. It's having perpetual money troubles or being in a destructive relationship or having constant fear about losing your job or being in stop-and-go commuter traffic every day.

The problem is, more and more of us are encountering chronic stress. In our instant-messaging, ever multitasking, chaotic world, we are forever rushing to get more and more done and stressing about everything from "downsizing" at work to terrorist attacks that can happen along the way. It's our hearts that ultimately pay the price.

For one thing, chronic stress makes us impatient, and impatience sends blood pressure skyward. In a study of 3,142 men and women who were followed for 15 years, researchers at Northwestern University found that people who said they usually felt pressed for time, ate too quickly, and got upset when they had to wait were twice as likely to develop hypertension as those who walked through life more relaxed.

Constant worrying can be even worse. In the landmark Brigham and Women's Hospital study of 37,000 nurses, researchers found that those who fretted the most about losing their jobs faced an almost twofold risk of having heart attacks compared with those who worried the least. Mental stress impairs the endothelium, the protective barrier that lines your blood vessels, paving the way for a series of inflammatory reactions that lead to fat and cholesterol buildup in the coronary arteries and ultimately—as the study above indicates—a heart attack.

Finally, stress can make you fat. Uncontrolled stress not only increases levels of the hormone cortisol, which directs fat storage straight to your waistline, it also makes you more likely to overeat, especially refined comfort foods, such as candy and chips, that trigger feel-good, tension-lowering hormones.

Your goal is to make small changes to maintain healthy tension while reducing excess stress.

Stress—Out!

Stress reduction is a billion-dollar industry, as consumers pour more and more money into self-help books, stone massages, scented candles, and Caribbean cruises, all in the name of relaxation. But the truth is that you don't have to spend a dime to soothe your stress, nor do you need tons of time. First, eat well and exercise to bolster your immunity and burn off built-up stress. When you maintain a healthy weight and overall good physical condition, you're much better equipped to deal with daily stress. Then practice a few of these mental tricks to stay calm and collected in the face of even the most hectic, harried day.

Focus and finish. Americans are obsessed with multitasking: Why just drive when you can also eat dinner and talk to your spouse on the phone? When you divide your attention three ways, nothing gets your full focus, leaving you frazzled and unsatisfied. Switch your thinking from "10 things at once" to "1 and done." Focus and finish each task at hand before moving on to the next. With your full attention, each job will take less time, and you'll feel a sense of control and accomplishment at the end of the day.

Take a news break. Boycott all news one day a week. If something *really* important happens, you'll hear about it, but you won't take your body through the excessive daily stress brought on by poring over the crimes and catastrophes from every corner of the world.

Shhh. Some forward-thinking companies have "quiet rooms" where employees can escape the whir of printers, telephones, fax machines, and pagers, if only for a minute. Set up your own silent space in your home where you can go to gather your thoughts when you're experiencing stimulation overload. It's surprising how well sitting there for just 30 seconds can help quell stress before it gets out of control.

Practice mindful meditation. Classic meditation, in which you try to clear your mind and sit silently for 10 to 20 minutes while repeating a phrase like "Om" is a scientifically proven stress reducer. There's just one problem: Few Americans actually do it. An easier alternative is mindful meditation, which you can do while walking down the street or washing your car. Simply focus your mind on what's happening in the immediate present. For instance, when washing your car, think of nothing but how the cool water bubbles up in the bucket, how the spray sounds as it breaks against the hood of your car, and how the water

runs in sheets, then beads in the sun. Then notice how much calmer you feel when the car is all clean. Practice mindful meditation once a day.

Laugh it up. In a study of 300 men and women, researchers at the University of Maryland found that people with heart disease were 40 percent less likely to laugh in a variety of situations than those of the same age without heart disease. Although more research is needed to understand the protective power of a good belly laugh, the researchers believe that stress reduction plays a major role. Rent *Caddyshack*, pick up a Calvin & Hobbes collection, or call a funny friend. Try to have a good laugh at least five times a day.

Take your time off. More than 30 percent of American workers fail to use all their vacation time each year. Time away to regenerate makes you a more productive worker and helps your heart. One government study showed that women who take two vacations a year are nearly eight times less likely to develop heart disease than those who take fewer. Planning vacations in advance ensures that (a) you'll take them; (b) everyone can plan for when you're gone; and (c) you always have something to look forward to.

See yourself succeed. Before you embark on a particularly stressful project, mentally rehearse it from beginning to end, advises cycling coach Bill Humphreys, who counsels athletes on how to stay cool under extreme pressure. "When you envision a task, you're mentally programming yourself to act through it," he says. "Then when you start, it's second nature." While you're at it, keep your self-talk positive. "Just by saying,

'I can do this,' you'll feel calmer and more confident than if you immediately start thinking 'Oh, no. I can't,'" says Humphreys.

Adopt a pet. Stress reduction is a good excuse to bring home a four-footed companion. Researchers at the State University of New York at Buffalo tested 48 stockbrokers already taking medication for high blood pressure in stressful situations, such as trying to calm a client who had lost $86,000 because of bad advice. Those who had pets had a systolic blood pressure rise from 120 to 126; those without a fluffy friend saw their systolic reading skyrocket from 120 to 148. Nothing calms like unconditional love.

Breathe deep. For instant calm in a stressful situation, stop and take four or five deep breaths, inhaling so your stomach rises. "Physiologically, it is practically impossible to not calm down when you're breathing slowly and deeply with your diaphragm," says panic researcher David F. Colvard, M.D., of Raleigh, North Carolina.

Tune in. Music hath charms to soothe the savage breast, or at the very least, bring down raging blood pressure during high-stress times. As proof, the Buffalo researchers tested 40 men and women who were about to undergo eye surgery, all of whom had elevated blood pressure in anticipation of the procedure. One group was given headphones and their choice of music to listen to; the others waited in silence. Within 5 minutes, the blood pressure levels of the music listeners dropped to normal and stayed there throughout the surgery. The tuneless volunteers had elevated blood pressure for the entire surgical experience. Store some mellow, upbeat music by your stereo to reach for when you're feeling tense.

Rub it out. Stress makes your muscles tense up, which reduces circulation and hampers the flow of both oxygen and nutrients. Massage helps loosen those muscles, relieve that built-up stress, and open the channels. For a simple self-massage, hold a tennis ball in your palm and roll it in a circular motion from the bottom of your neck to your shoulders as well as your thighs, hips, and calves, the soles of your feet, and anywhere else you feel tension.

Don't take the bait. Stress is your *reaction* to external events, not the events themselves. While you often can't control an external event, you *can* control your reaction. The next time something happens that typically angers you or stresses you out, pause and ask yourself, "Is this worth getting upset over? Will feeling stressed out accomplish anything?" Often, the answer to both questions is no. That awareness goes a long way toward diminishing stressful reactions to challenging situations.

Get your z's. Fatigue makes you less able to cope with stressful situations. When you are well rested, you are more resilient and better able to deal with everyday events. Shoot for 8 hours a night.

Cry it out. Ever notice how much better you feel after a good cry? That's because tears flush out harmful chemicals produced during stress and release pent-up negative energy. If all else fails, let the tears flow. You'll feel better when you're done.

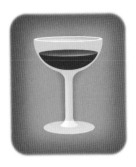

Alcohol
(in Moderation)

WE ALL HAVE our alcohol habits. Some of us like wine with dinner, and others enjoy a cold brew while watching the game. Some choose not to drink at all, while others drink too much. People have been indulging in fermented beverages for 10,000 years and have been debating their health benefits (and detriments) for nearly as long.

The fact is that alcohol is both medicinal and poisonous. The distinction between its Jekyll-and-Hyde natures lies in the dose. Consumed in moderation—that's no more than one to two drinks a day—alcohol delivers a host of benefits. Studies show that not only do temperate drinkers enjoy longer lives than both heavy drinkers and teetotalers, they also have significantly better heart health.

Multiple landmark studies, collectively including more than 750,000 men and women, show that moderate drinking lowers the risk of heart disease, heart attack, and/or cardiovascular-related death by 30 to 40 percent. Sensible drinkers also tend to have healthy lifestyle habits. They're more likely than nondrinkers or heavy drinkers to maintain a healthy weight, get 7 to 8 hours of sleep nightly, and exercise regularly, according to surveys. Anecdotally, they also report enjoying rich, relaxed social lives. In short, they have happy hearts—emotionally and physically.

The opposite can be said of those who drink too much. Ethanol, the active ingredient in alcoholic beverages, impairs cognitive function and wreaks havoc on all the body's organs when taken in excess. Heavy drinking can contribute to or directly cause high blood pressure, obesity, cardiomyopathy (dangerous inflammation of the heart), heart failure, cardiac arrhythmia (irregular heartbeat), and sudden cardiac death. That's not even considering other risks, such as automobile accidents and alcoholism, that are commonly associated with overindulgence.

Because the risks can far outweigh the benefits, you definitely should not start drinking if you don't already imbibe. If you currently enjoy alcohol judiciously, however, there are ways to get more heart benefits from your beverages.

The Great Grape

Whether you prefer martinis, merlot, or Miller Lite, all alcohol provides some cardio protection. A report from the Health Professionals Follow-Up Study of more than 38,000 men showed that moderate drinkers had healthier hearts regardless of their drink choice. That's because, in proper doses, alcohol raises levels of good HDL cholesterol while altering factors in the blood so it's less likely to clot.

Although any drink is good, if you want the healthiest toast, wine may be best, according to several decades' worth of research. By now, you've heard of the "French paradox"—the ironic discovery that although the French smoke cigarettes and consume a saturated-fat-laden diet, they are still 2½ times less likely to develop heart disease than more health-conscious Americans. Researchers credited their heart health to their penchant for rich red wines, particularly since studies have also found that wine-drinking nations have lower rates of heart disease than beer- or liquor-drinking countries.

Aspirin and Alcohol Don't Mix

If your doctor has advised you to take aspirin for heart protection, don't drink. The FDA warns that the combination can damage the stomach lining and even cause stomach bleeding. Don't stop taking aspirin without talking to your doctor.

Although we've since identified other factors in French life, such as daily physical activity and a relaxed lifestyle, that contribute to cardiovascular resilience, there's no question that wine contains compounds that can fight the heart attackers on every front.

At the forefront of wine's artery-clearing arsenal is a family of antioxidant compounds called polyphenols, including a flavonoid called quercetin and the compound resveratrol, both of which apparently help prevent the body's dangerous LDL cholesterol from oxidizing. This makes cholesterol less likely to stick to artery walls. Both quercetin and resveratrol also work like WD-40 in the bloodstream, making blood cells less likely to stick together and clot.

Now under investigation is another cardio-friendly army of compounds called saponins. Found in the waxy skin of grapes, they appear to promote heart health by binding to cholesterol and preventing its absorption in the blood. They may also help reduce harmful inflammation.

Think When You Drink

If you choose to indulge, why not choose wisely? The following tips will help you enjoy alcohol while also helping your heart.

Go for gusto. Sorry, chardonnay fans, but for health benefits, white wines pale in comparison to their ruby-hued counterparts. That's because white wines are traditionally made without grape skins (or the mashed mixture containing the skins is removed early in the process), which is where the most protective compounds are found. When choosing a red, look for full-bodied, robust varieties, which harbor the most heart-healthy chemicals. Three with the best bouquets overall are cabernet sauvignon, petite sirah, and merlot. For the highest saponin counts, reach for red zinfandel, syrah, pinot noir, or cabernet sauvignon.

Drink with dinner. Some studies suggest that the cholesterol-conquering, anticlotting powers of wine are most pronounced when you drink it as part of your main meal. A bonus: Wine is a time-honored digestive aid. Scientists at Tripler Army Medical Center in Honolulu have found that wine is more effective at wiping out harmful food-borne bacteria than bismuth subsalicylate (otherwise known as Pepto-Bismol).

Take your supplements. Alcohol blocks the absorption of folate and inactivates it in the bloodstream. That's bad because this B vitamin helps rid the body of homocysteine and helps build DNA in newly generated cells. Although moderate alcohol consumption as part of a healthy diet shouldn't pose a problem, few people eat enough leafy greens and other folate-rich foods to begin with. Researchers recommend that people who drink alcohol get 600 micrograms of folate a day. You can ensure that you reach that mark by popping a daily multivitamin that includes folic acid (the supplement form of folate).

Double Trouble

If you drink, you probably drink more than you think. That's because most people really don't know what a serving looks like, or that if they drink at restaurants and bars, they're being given a serving and a half or even a double serving with each drink.

A drink is considered 12 ounces of beer; 4 ounces of wine (half a standard drinking cup); 1.5 ounces of 80-proof spirits, such as gin or vodka; or 1 ounce of 100-proof spirits, such as some kinds of whiskey and bourbon. If you don't know what those amounts look like, pour the proper serving into a measuring cup, then transfer it to your favorite drinking glass.

Get benefits without the booze. You can get all the benefits of grapes without the alcohol buzz by drinking purple grape juice or even nonalcoholic wine, which contains the same active ingredients as real wine minus the alcohol. Remember that alcohol provides its own heart protection, though, so ethanol-free drinks won't deliver quite the same healthy cardiovascular kick.

Watch the mixers. Many ingredients in mixed drinks are filled with sugar and high in calories. Opt for club soda, water, or unsweetened juice instead of sugary sodas, sweet liqueurs, or premade mixes for drinks like margaritas or bloody Marys.

Drink less—more often. It should go without saying: Drinking an average of 1 to 2 drinks a day does not mean drinking nothing all week and having 12 on Saturday and Sunday. Research shows that men who drink a little every day have lower risks of heart attack than those who drink more once or twice a week.

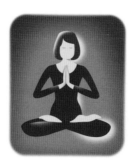

Yoga

STAND UP. REALLY, stand up. Inhale deeply and reach for the sky, as high as you can. Next, slowly blow your breath out, sweeping your arms past your sides and bending toward the floor as you empty your lungs. Draw fresh air into your lungs and slowly roll back up to a standing position, arms by your sides. Feels good, doesn't it?

You can sit down now.

What you just did was sample the simple science of yoga—moving your body to fend off sitting disease while clearing your mind to nurture a peaceful, happy, healthy heart.

Unlike Western medicine, which takes the Jiffy Lube approach to wellness by directing you to a fix-it specialist for each of your broken parts (Bunions? See a podiatrist. Depression? That's a psychiatrist's job!), traditional Eastern medicine uses holistic systems such as yoga to treat your mind and body as one.

Developed 5,000 years ago in India, yoga reached American shores with immigrants back in the 1800s. Only in recent decades, though, has our faster-moving, increasingly stressed population embraced this exercise that's more serene than sweat, more meditative than muscle. Today in the United States, more than 15 million people include yoga in their regular fitness routines. Its advocates range from Madonna to Sandra Day O'Connor and from NFL running backs to Wall Street brokers.

Although some people focus their practice more behind—striving for the coveted firm "yoga butt"—than inward, scientific evidence from the past 10 years shows that this traditional-yet-trendy, mind-body medicine can relieve symptoms of chronic diseases such as cancer, arthritis, and yes, heart disease. Even hospitals are getting in on the act. At New York Presbyterian Hospital and Cedars-Sinai Medical Center in Los Angeles, cardiologists routinely steer patients into programs that offer yoga as part of their preventive and rehabilitative care.

Disease Reversal

Internationally renowned heart disease researcher Dean Ornish, M.D., of the Preventive Medicine Research Institute in Sausalito, California, may have been the first Western physician to place yoga alongside diet and exercise at the foundation of a heart-healthy lifestyle. In his most cited study in 1990, Dr. Ornish tested 48 men and women with medically documented coronary heart disease. The doctor assigned 28 participants to a lifestyle regimen that included yoga, group counseling, and an extremely low-fat vegetarian diet. The rest received their usual care and continued their regular lifestyle habits.

Hooked?

Once you get a taste of yoga, you may find yourself craving a full course. Investing more time will help you reap even more benefits. Yoga builds strength, as well as increasing flexibility and promoting a sense of calm. Luckily, yoga information is easy to find. Bookstores have lots of great guides; almost all gyms and senior centers offer classes; videos are available at the library; yoga magazines are on newsstands; and, of course, the Internet has an overwhelming amount of information.

After a year, those in Dr. Ornish's test group actually had clearer, more supple arteries—indicating that their heart disease was reversing—while the arteries of those in the control group continued to clog and harden. Eight years later, he published a follow-up study showing that 80 percent of 194 men and women with heart disease were able to avoid bypass surgery by following a similar lifestyle intervention program that included yoga.

Although the lion's share of his colleagues credited the spartan, zero-saturated-fat food plan with bulldozing built-up plaque, Dr. Ornish steadfastly argues that adherence to yoga is as strongly correlated with reductions in artery blockage as is adherence to the diet.

During a 2003 study, a research team in India tested 113 men and women, ages 35 to 70, with documented coronary artery disease. They placed 71 in a yoga lifestyle program, which included stress management, exercise, and a plant-based diet, while the remaining volunteers took heart medications and followed a more typical Western medicine prescription of diet and lifestyle tweaks. One year later, the yoga group had fared much better, averaging a 23 percent drop in cholesterol levels compared with only a 4 percent reduction among the med-taking volunteers. What's more, 44 percent of the yoga participants showed reversals of their heart disease, and artery hardening was stopped in its tracks for 47 percent—significantly greater improvements than those in the control group.

Sweet Slumber

You can do yoga anytime, but we recommend it before bedtime as a way to quiet the stresses of the day. In fact, you can actually do yoga *in bed*. The following four introductory yoga poses are good for increasing circulation around the heart and promoting relaxation. And yes, you can do them on your mattress, in your PJs, before turning down the covers and calling it a night. Hold each pose for at least 30 seconds.

COBRA POSE

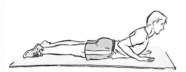

LIE FACEDOWN with your feet together, your toes pointed behind you, and your hands palms down just in front of your shoulders. Lift your chin and gently raise your head and chest so your torso is supported on your forearms. Be sure to keep your shoulders down and back, not hunched up by your ears. Remember to breathe deeply throughout. People sometimes hold their breath during this move, which is not good if you have existing heart disease.

SPINAL TWIST

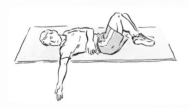

LIE ON YOUR BACK with your knees bent, your feet flat, and your arms at your sides. Slowly lower your knees to the left while simultaneously extending your arms to the right as far as comfortably possible. Keep your shoulders in contact with the floor or bed. Repeat on the other side, holding each position for 15 seconds.

PRAYER POSE

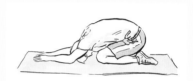

KNEEL with the tops of your feet on the floor or bed and your toes pointed behind you. Sit back onto your heels, then lower your chest to your thighs. Extend your arms and rest your palms and forehead on the floor (or as close as comfortably possible).

CORPSE POSE

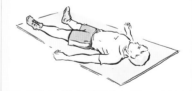

LIE ON YOUR BACK with your arms at your sides and your palms facing up. Place your heels slightly apart and allow your feet to fall naturally to the sides. Starting with your feet, progressively contract or flex and then relax all of your muscles (i.e., your toes, then your ankles, calves, knees, and so on to the top of your head). When you're finished, relax, breathe deeply, and—nighty-night.

Fight-or-Flight Deactivated

While there's no denying that diet is a powerful component of the "yoga lifestyle," the ability of this flowing, serene exercise to defuse stress is probably yoga's most potent power in battling heart disease. We've all heard of the fight-or-flight response, which occurs when, at the slightest whiff of threat, your body's Fort Knoxian personal security system gushes adrenaline and cortisol into your bloodstream to mobilize fat from your body's stores to fuel your muscles—and your escape. The problem is, in modern society, you're more likely to face an angry boss than a charging buffalo, so instead of fighting or fleeing, you're left stewing in that toxic self-defense cocktail. The result: elevated blood pressure, higher cholesterol, and an increased likelihood of blood clots.

Now for some good news. Just as your body is equipped with a punch-and-run reflex during times of perceived danger, it also has a pretty good peacetime plan, known as the relaxation response, which gives your battle-weary nervous system some much-needed R&R. The catch: Like a day spent with your mind wrapped up in a novel and your toes nestled in warm sand, the relaxation response doesn't just happen during everyday chaotic life. You have to pursue it—and yoga is one of the best paths you can take.

As you draw in deep belly breaths and release built-up tension by extending your limbs through their full range of motion, focusing your thoughts on each pose, you flip the switch that deactivates the fight-or-flight system and engages the relaxation response. Your heartbeat slows and your blood pressure drops. Over time, if you practice regularly, you can even lower the "alert level" of your autonomic nervous system so that you're walking around more relaxed all the time.

Relaxation doesn't just happen during everyday chaotic life. You have to pursue it.

Like standard stretching, yoga also increases circulation and improves blood supply to the heart. With better blood flow, your heart doesn't have to work as hard to deliver fresh nutrients and oxygen to your organs and muscles. By entering a relaxed state, you also increase your coronary blood flow by decreasing artery constriction.

As a side benefit, regular yoga stretching lengthens muscles and connective tissues, improving your flexibility and range of motion so you can enjoy heart-healthy aerobic and strengthening activities with less muscle soreness and chronic aches and pains.

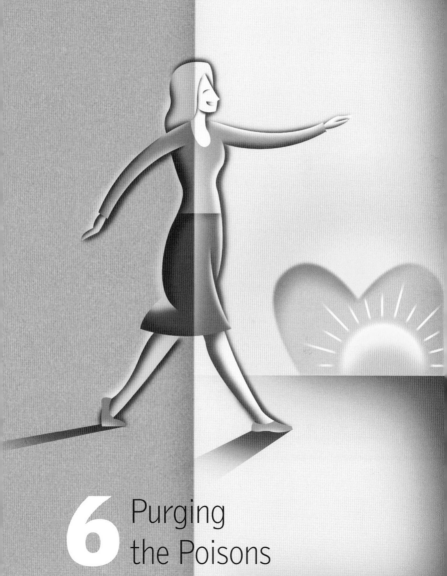

6 Purging the Poisons

*Germs and toxic chemicals are pervasive
in our lives. Ignoring them is easy
—and risky. Being mindful of
them is also easy—and will
protect your heart
and your life.*

Heal with Clean Living

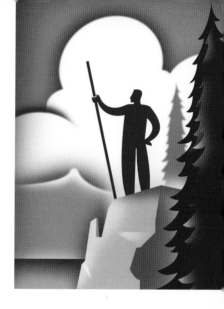

THEY SAY THAT CLEANLINESS is next to godliness. That's up to the theologians to debate, but we can tell you with absolute certainty that cleanliness *is* next to healthiness. Like your car, lawn mower, and household appliances, your body works best when you keep it clean. Your heart especially appreciates a tidy home, free of germs, bacteria, dirt, and general artery-clogging grime.

Nonsmokers, for instance, can live a full 15 years longer than those who light up all day, day after day. Shielding yourself from flu viruses can slash your risk of heart disease by a fifth or more. Even just brushing the fuzzy coat of plaque from your teeth twice a day may prevent a future heart attack!

Here's another inescapable fact of life: As much as we may like the end result, most of us simply do not like to clean—and that goes for our lifestyles as much as our living rooms. In a culture that celebrates fatty food, booze, and tobacco consumption as grownup entertainment, clean living gets a bad rap for not being much fun. But you don't have to be a killjoy to live a clean, heart-healthy life. We promise.

Purge the Poisons

Some of this—such as the case against cigarette smoking—is advice you've undoubtedly heard before, but many of the revelations linking everyday environmental offenders to heart disease will probably surprise you. Back in "Eating Outside the Box," we talked about how additives, man-made fats, and processed foods are poisons for your heart. In this section, we'll talk about the nonfood toxins that affect it. You'll discover how the smallest steps, such as using mouthwash or getting a simple shot, can help keep your arteries clear and your heart happy and healthy for years to come. Detailed in the pages that follow are a few simple steps for purging heart-damaging poisons, including:

• **Keep a clean mouth.** The way to your heart is through your mouth. No, not by way of your stomach—by way of your arteries. Believe it or not, bacteria from sticky dental plaque can seep through infected gums and wreak havoc in your circulatory system. Having clean teeth and healthy gums will really give you something to smile about.

• **Scrub your hands.** Germs are everywhere. Using soap and water stops them from getting into your eyes, nose, or mouth, where they can set up shop and pave the way for infection and heart-damaging inflammation. Practicing good personal hygiene fights more than colds; it can keep heart disease at bay as well.

• **Get your shots.** Being vaccinated against common ailments such as the flu can slash your risk of being hospitalized with heart disease–related problems and drastically reduce your risk of having a heart attack if you're already in a high-risk category. What's more, vaccinations are often free—and can help you avoid being laid up in bed.

Environmental pollution—in the air you breathe, the water you drink, even the food you eat—can greatly affect heart health.

• **Filter your air and water.** Environmental pollution is a newly recognized heart disease risk. It's not surprising that the air you breathe, the water you drink, and the food you eat can greatly affect your heart health, particularly if they're contaminated. But you don't have to live in a bubble to protect that precious pump of yours. Just take a few simple steps to filter out the worst offenders.

• **Ban tobacco.** Okay, this one may seem a little killjoyish if you're a lifelong puffer who savors every smoke break, but tobacco is public enemy number one among pollutants that cause cardiovascular disease. Smokers have a 70 percent greater chance of dying from heart disease than people who don't use tobacco. Lighting up not only damages your own heart and arteries, but every time you expose someone else to cigarette smoke, it accelerates hardening of the arteries for them, too. The longer you smoke, the higher your risk; conversely, the sooner you quit, the faster your heart heals. Quitting is hard, but with modern medicines and nicotine replacement strategies, it's anything but impossible. If you care about your heart, you must stop smoking. Your doctor can help, and if you follow the strategies in the following pages, you can start living smoke-free today. You'll enjoy life more than ever.

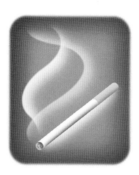

Tobacco

IF DOCTORS KNEW a few centuries ago what we know about tobacco today, this chapter probably wouldn't even exist. Back then, medical experts thought tobacco was *good* for you. In 1571, one Spanish doctor even wrote a book claiming that tobacco could cure 36 different diseases. For hundreds of years, American Indians used tobacco for both religious and medicinal reasons. The deadly plant from the nightshade family was used to dress wounds, kill pain, and commune with nature.

We've come a long way, baby!

After 40 years of warnings from the U.S. Surgeon General, today we know that rather than healing, tobacco use—specifically, smoking cigarettes—shaves an average of 10 years off users' lives. It's true: A 50-year study of 34,439 British doctors by the now 91-year-old researcher who first connected cigarettes to lung cancer in the 1950s linked smoking to 25 diseases and a steep rise in mortality—shortening life expectancy by a decade. Among men born in the 1920s who became regular smokers, two-thirds died from their habits. Recent reports from the Centers for Disease Control and Prevention are even graver. Based on data collected from 1995 to 1999, it's estimated that adult male smokers lost an average of 13.2 years of life and females an astonishing 14.5 years.

Smoking is especially hard on your heart. Smokers have a 70 percent greater chance of dying from heart disease than nonsmokers. If you're under 40, you're five times more likely to have a heart attack if you smoke than if you don't, according to a Finnish study of 4,047 men and women. Smoking cigarettes elevates your heart rate, raises your blood pressure, increases the clotting factors in your blood, depletes good HDL cholesterol, increases dangerous triglycerides, and damages the linings of your blood vessels. That's not even considering its role in related vascular disease, such as carotid artery blockages, stroke, impotence, and chronic obstructive pulmonary disease. In the end, more smokers die from tobacco-related heart disease than from lung cancer.

Every Puff You Take

Each drag from a cigarette dumps more than 4,000 chemicals into your bloodstream. About 50 of them are known to cause cancer, but that's over the long term. With every inhalation, you immediately breathe in two potent poisons—nicotine and carbon monoxide—that together create a burden that's more than most hearts can bear.

Nicotine is the reason most smokers light up. It creates a pleasant, relaxed feeling of euphoria. Ironically, it's also a highly toxic stimulant that would probably kill you if you actually absorbed all the nicotine in just two cigarettes. In reality, you absorb only a fraction of the chemical from each butt, but it's still enough to rev your heart rate into unhealthy territory. Carbon monoxide, the poisonous emission from automobile engines, is also formed when tobacco burns. When you breathe it into your lungs, it replaces the oxygen in your red blood cells, so your heart has to beat that much harder to get oxygen and nutrients from your blood. Making matters worse, the buildup of fat deposits caused by exposure to nicotine and carbon monoxide makes your blood vessels

and arteries narrower, further limiting blood supply to your heart.

Over time, you can count on having blocked blood vessels and arteries, which can lead to permanent heart damage. In turn, the lack of oxygen for your over-stressed heart paves the way for a heart attack. The longer you smoke and the more cigarettes you burn through, the higher your risk.

Put Out the Fire

While most of the news surrounding tobacco use is grim, there is a silver lining to this cloud of smoke. You can stop the harmful effects in their tracks and even eventually reverse the damage by taking a hard line against tobacco. No matter how long you've smoked, your risk of heart attack decreases just 24 hours after you quit. After a year, your tobacco-related risk of heart disease is half that of a current smoker's, and 15 years after you crush your last butt, your risk drops to the level of someone who's never lit up. Here's what you need to know about ridding tobacco from your life.

It takes inspiration. So, you've just read all about how terrible tobacco is for you—news you get on the side panel of your cigarette pack every time you pick one up. Most smokers know smoking is bad for them, but that knowledge doesn't inspire them to quit. Those smokers benefit from finding external motivation, perhaps quitting for people they love, such as their children or grandchildren. Think about what cherished life events you might miss if your life were cut short by 10 or 15 years. The birth of a grandchild? A grandchild's wedding?

My Quit-Smoking Contract

I, _____, will quit smoking on _____ (date). From that day on,
I will be a nonsmoker, free of the physical, mental, social, and economic burdens of tobacco use.

I am quitting smoking for myself, but also for (list loved ones)_____
_____

When I feel the need to smoke, I will use the following strategies to overcome the craving.
_____
_____

If I need support, I will call _____

After three months smoke-free, I will reward myself with _____

    My six-month reward will be _____

    My nine-month reward will be _____

    I will celebrate one year of smoke-free living with _____

Signature: _____ Witness: _____

Whom will you miss, or who will miss you most, if you die more than a decade prematurely? Quit for them.

Your doctor can help. Although it's perfectly legal, tobacco can be as addictive as illegal street drugs such as cocaine or heroin. It can take two or three tries, or more, to quit for good. Involving your doctor improves your chances. Studies have shown that about 70 percent of smokers want to quit and that those who have the support of their health care providers are most successful. But don't count on your doctor to broach this sensitive subject. Only half of smokers who see physicians have ever been urged to quit, according to surveys. Take the initiative. Tell your doctor you want to quit and ask for help.

Substitutions rarely work. Contrary to popular opinion, switching to "lighter" cigarettes will not protect your health or help you quit. For one thing, scientists have found that light cigarettes can yield higher levels of nicotine than what's listed on their labels. People also tend to puff harder, longer, and more often on light cigarettes to get the desired nicotine "fix." Likewise, smoking cigars or a pipe is a poor cessation strategy, since you still absorb nicotine into your bloodstream and probably still inhale at least some of every puff.

But exercise does. Regular exercise can help you quit smoking by burning off stress hormones, so you feel less of an urge to smoke, and producing feel-good brain chemicals to help reduce the uncomfortable effects of nicotine withdrawal. A Gallup Poll found that smokers who exercised were twice as likely to quit as their sedentary counterparts. Daily exercise can also help you avoid the dreaded 5- to 10-pound weight gain commonly associated with kicking the habit.

Chewing tobacco is a problem, too. Smokeless tobacco, or "chew," is not a safe alternative to smoking. True, you don't get carbon monoxide from chewing tobacco, but you still get high levels of nicotine, which increase your risk of high blood pressure and heart disease. It also elevates your risk of devastating oral cancer. If you need something to do with your mouth, consider chewing sugarless gum instead.

Good influences help. Hanging out with smokers not only makes it harder to quit because of the ever-present temptation, it also hurts your heart to breathe the air they pollute. Persistent exposure to cigarette smoke, either at home or on the job, nearly doubles your risk of having a heart attack even if you don't smoke, according to a landmark 10-year study of more than 32,000 women. Another recent analysis combining the results of 18 studies that involved more than half a million men and women showed that regular exposure to passive tobacco smoke raises risk of heart disease by 25 percent. The American Heart Association now blames as many as 40,000 heart disease deaths a year on secondhand smoke. If you socialize with smokers, do so in nonsmoking establishments, where they can puff outdoors. If you live with a smoker, take the ashtray outside and keep it there. Establish a nonsmoking house today.

How to Quit Smoking —for Good

The great American wit Mark Twain once remarked, "Quitting smoking is easy. I've done it a thousand times." No truer words were ever spoken on the subject. Nicotine is highly addictive and *very* hard for some people to shake. Once you're hooked, cutting back or quitting can lead to a laundry list of withdrawal symptoms, such as irritability, depression, frustration, anger, restlessness, headache, fatigue, increased appetite, trouble concentrating, and sleep disturbances. Despite the unpleasant transition period, however, half of all adult smokers have managed to quit, with more kicking the habit every day. Here are the top seven strategies of successful quitters.

1. Set a date

Quitting smoking takes mental (and physical) preparation. Pick a "quit date" within the next month and circle it on your calendar. Between now and then, set the stage for your smoke-free life. This is an exciting time, so be enthusiastic. Stock up on sugarless gum, baby carrots, and hard candy. The night before the big day, throw out all your cigarettes, ashtrays, matches, lighters, and other smoking supplies. You're a nonsmoker now; you don't need them.

2. Make an announcement

Tell your friends, family, and coworkers about your quit day. Don't be embarrassed if you've made this proclamation before. Remind them that it often takes repeated attempts for quitting to "stick" and ask for their help in making this attempt the last one.

3. Establish support

Studies show that having a strong support network increases your chances of successfully quitting smoking. Nicotine Anonymous offers on-call support, booklets, and other helpful information on breaking the tobacco habit. You can find a meeting near you at www.nicotine-anonymous.org, or contact your nearest medical facility. Almost all hospitals offer smoking cessation programs. Consider working with a group for the first three months—the time frame in which most relapses occur.

4. Create diversions

Smoking is a pastime as much as an addiction. You smoke for something to do during breaks at work, while driving your car, and during quiet evenings at home. Once you quit, you'll feel that something is missing during these times. Fill the space with other activity. Sip water and sing along to a favorite CD while you drive. Take short walks instead of coffee breaks. Choose hands-on activities such as crocheting or refinishing furniture to do as you wind down in the evening. You'll miss cigarettes less if you keep busy.

5. Consider nicotine replacement

Many smokers successfully quit cold turkey, but you can double your chances of success (provided you also adjust your behavior as suggested above) by using some form of nicotine replacement during the initial adjustment period. Many forms of nicotine replacement products are available both over the counter and by prescription, including gum, inhalers, nasal sprays, and patches. Increase your odds of succeeding even more (by 58 percent, according to studies) by combining nicotine replacement therapy with an antidepressant drug called bupropion (Zyban).

Nicotine replacement products work by relieving symptoms of withdrawal without providing the "buzz" that keeps smokers hooked. Because nicotine can be extremely toxic in high doses, it's essential that you use these products only as directed—and never smoke while using them. The combination can be deadly.

6. Avoid triggers

Drinking and smoking go together like peanut butter and jelly. Switch to water, juices, or low-cal sodas instead of alcohol, especially during that very vulnerable initial quitting period of two to three months. Later on, you'll be able to handle a drink with more confidence. But remember, alcohol always lowers inhibitions, so you'll have to remain vigilant. Some people have a strong coffee-cigarette association as well. In that case, find an alternate source of caffeine, such as tea, which is less likely to trigger a craving (provided you weren't a tea drinker–cigarette smoker to begin with).

7. Take 10

When you feel the urge to light up—and you will—look at your watch and give yourself 10 minutes. During that time, take full, deep breaths as you would if you were drawing on a cigarette. Deep breathing will fill your lungs with clean, smoke-free air and trigger a relaxation response. By the time 10 minutes is up, the acute urge to smoke will have passed, and you'll be better able to move past the craving.

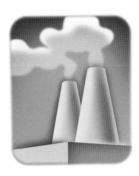

Pollution

IT'S COMMON SENSE, really, but only recently has research confirmed it: Air pollution causes heart disease.

That's not some alarmist warning from a fringe environmental group; it's a statement from the American Heart Association (AHA). In fact, the AHA says, air pollution is even worse for your heart than it is for your lungs. In a study that analyzed data from a survey of 500,000 adults, epidemiologists from Brigham Young University in Provo, Utah, found that air pollution in U.S. cities causes twice as many deaths from heart disease as it does from lung cancer and other respiratory ailments.

"This is a serious public health problem due to the enormous number of people affected and because exposure to air pollution occurs over an entire lifetime," reports Robert Book of the University of Michigan in Ann Arbor, who helped the AHA write the warning statement.

High Traffic Clogs Arteries

The pollution risk is from what scientists call combustion-related fine particulate matter. That's a fancy name for soot. It seems the black stuff that clogs chimneys also clogs arteries—and it's not coming just from fireplaces. Soot is emitted by cars, trucks, factories, and coal-fired power plants. When you breathe it in, the particulate matter irritates your airways and triggers an inflammatory response, which, like all inflammation, accelerates plaque buildup and narrowing of the arteries.

The Environmental Protection Agency (EPA) estimates that each year, 60,000 people in the United States alone die from this kind of particulate air pollution. Not surprisingly, high-traffic areas pose the greatest danger. An eight-year study of 5,000 adults showed that people who lived near heavily trafficked roads were more likely to die from heart disease–related conditions than those who were farther from the exhaust-belching flow of cars and trucks.

Even heart-healthy activities such as jogging or cycling can be harmful when done in areas with poor air quality. In a study of 45 women who exercised regularly in the Helsinki area, Finnish researchers found that when pollution levels were high, the volunteers had significantly higher levels of ischemia (decreased blood flow to the heart), even two days after exercising, than when the air was clearer. Their resting heart rates also increased after exposure to pollution, from an average of 61 beats per minute to 90.

Although air pollution hurts everyone, older adults and people with existing conditions such as heart disease and diabetes are at particularly high risk.

Breathe Better

Aside from writing to your elected officials, driving cleaner cars, and supporting clean air movements, there's not much you can do to change the air you breathe (except move to the country). There are, however, several small steps you can take to greatly limit your heart's exposure to the damaging effects of dirty air.

Check the index before you exercise. In 1997, the EPA introduced the National Ambient Air Quality Standards (NAAQS) to spread the word about air quality issues. The index provides air breathability measurements for more than 150 cities, based on the levels of ozone and particulates in the air. The EPA also issues alerts when air pollution hits dangerously high levels. If you live in a highly populated area, check your local newspaper for either an Air Quality Index (AQI) or Pollution Standards Index (PSI) before you head out to exercise, especially in the summer, when pollution tends to be at its worst. When the

Something in the Air...and the Water...and...

Unfortunately, pollution is pervasive. It's not just in the air we breathe but also in the water we drink and sometimes the food we eat. These other environmental offenders can also be hard on your heart. In a recent study of 2,125 men and women ages 40 and over, researchers at the Johns Hopkins Medical Institutions in Baltimore found that on average, those with periph-

eral artery disease had 14 percent higher blood levels of lead and 16 percent higher blood levels of cadmium. Both pollutants can be found in air, food, and water (cadmium is also present in cigarette smoke). Other studies have suggested that high blood levels of mercury from eating too much highly contaminated fish may elevate heart disease risk as well.

Limit your exposure to harmful chemicals: Use water filters (such as Brita) either on the tap or in a special pitcher to eliminate contaminants in your drinking water. Follow the smart fish-eating guidelines on page 105, and limit your use of and exposure to known toxic substances such as pesticides, gasoline, and charcoal.

number climbs above 100, pollution is high. When it's above 200, stick to indoor exercise. Daily updates are also available on the EPA Web site, www.epa.gov/airnow.

Avoid rush hour. Even if the air in your area tends to be clean, avoid exercising at rush hour, when vehicle emissions are highest. Your best bet for avoiding sooty air: exercise in the early morning.

Stay away from smokers. The good news is that more bars, restaurants, and other public places throughout the country are banning smoking on their premises. The bad news: Exposure to secondhand smoke from just a single cigarette each day speeds the development of atherosclerosis. When someone lights up near you, excuse yourself until he's finished.

Filter with ferns. Good insulation and tightly sealed windows can save you cash on your heating bills, but they can wreak havoc with your home's air quality, especially when combined with recycled forced-air heat during winter months. Improve your air quality with some potted plants. Houseplants, especially ferns, spider plants, and rubber plants, work like air filters and create a calming ambience.

Eat your antioxidants. Antioxidant nutrients, such as vitamins C and E and beta-carotene, have been shown to protect your heart and lungs from the ill effects of pollution-induced free radical damage. But don't rely on supplements. The best sources come in the natural packages of fruits and vegetables. Following the 30-Minutes-A-Day Eating Plan and using the recipes in the 30-Minutes-A-Day Plan Workbook will provide protection.

Use your nose. When exercising in less-than-ideal air conditions, breathe through your nose as much as possible. Unlike your mouth, your nose is equipped with fine hairs that help filter the air before it reaches your lungs.

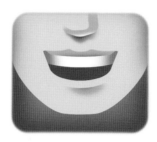

Tooth Plaque

HERE'S A SOBERING fact to chew on: People with chronic bacterial infections of the gums are nearly twice as likely to have fatal heart attacks as those with healthy gums. That's right. Evidence is mounting that brushing and flossing do more than give you a pretty smile: They can also save your life.

In a University of Minnesota study of more than 700 men and women with no history of heart disease, researchers found a direct relationship between missing teeth (an indicator of serious dental disease) and plaque buildup in the arteries. Other studies have linked periodontal (gum) disease with increased resting heart rate, abnormal electrocardiograms, and poor blood sugar control—all symptoms of or contributors to heart disease.

University of Michigan researchers who studied 320 U.S. veterans went so far as to conclude that dental disease was a larger risk factor for heart disease than being overweight, having high cholesterol, not exercising, or smoking. Talk about little habits, like brushing and flossing, adding up to great big heart health gains!

Gumming Up Your Arteries

We've intuitively known that bad teeth equal bad health for centuries—hence the advice not to look a gift horse in the mouth (back in the day, horses also had tattoos on their gums indicating their breeding history). It's been only recently, though, that we've identified the scientific connection: inflammation.

"Anything that causes low-grade inflammation, like chronic gum disease, may accelerate arteriosclerosis," says Robert Bonow, M.D., president of the American

Heart Association. The theory is that bacteria from dental plaque seep into the bloodstream through inflamed gums and produce enzymes that make blood platelets more sticky and likely to clot, contributing to hardening of the arteries and heart disease.

Brush Up on Heart Health

The good news is that this is a risk factor you can easily control. Here's what to do.

Brush for two. Put a kitchen timer on the bathroom sink. Set it for 2 minutes and, holding your toothbrush as you would a pencil, use gentle, circular strokes to brush your teeth at a 45-degree angle to your gums. Brush until the timer dings, hitting all surfaces of the teeth—front, back, and top. Tooth brushing reduces levels of all harmful bacteria in your mouth, especially *Streptococcus sanguis*, which has been shown to induce blood clots and hardening of the arteries in rabbits. Brush twice a day, in the morning and before bed. Replace your toothbrush every six months.

Develop a daily flossing ritual. An astonishing 85 percent of us fail to floss daily. Tie a bow of floss around the handle of your toothbrush as a reminder to clean between your teeth. Using about 18 inches of waxed floss, wind the majority around your left middle finger and the rest around your right middle finger, leaving a few inches in between. Gently maneuver the floss between your teeth and rub it up and down along the sides of each tooth, especially under the gum line. If flossing is difficult, try a floss holder or ask your dentist about interdental devices (tiny brushes) that can make the job easier.

Gum Disease Symptoms

You can have periodontal disease and not know it, so see your dentist regularly even if your teeth are healthy. Also, know the warning signs of gum disease:

- Gums that bleed easily
- Red, swollen, tender gums
- Gums that have pulled away from the teeth
- Persistent bad breath or a bad taste in your mouth
- Permanent teeth that are loose or separating from each other
- Any change in the way your teeth fit together when you bite
- Any change in the fit of partial dentures

Brush 'n' rinse. Two daily 30-second rinses with an antibacterial mouthwash can reduce tooth plaque by 20 percent, so swish some Listerine!

Book in advance. Set up appointments for professional cleanings twice a year, or every three months if you have heart disease. Always tell your dentist what medications you take, since some, like high blood pressure pills and oral contraceptives, can increase your risk of gum disease.

Stimulate saliva. A dry mouth increases dental decay. Ask your dentist about using sugar-free gum or candy or special rinses to stimulate saliva flow.

Use antibiotics, if necessary. People with preexisting heart conditions, especially valve defects, are at risk for a serious heart infection following dental procedures. Ask your doctor if you need to take antibiotics before having dental work done.

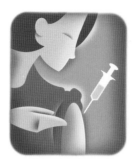

Viruses and Bacteria

WHAT IF THERE were a cheap, safe, 5-minute treatment that could significantly decrease your risk of being hospitalized for heart disease and stroke and reduce your overall risk of dying by as much as 50 percent? You'd waste no time signing up! But do you get your flu shot every year? If not, you're missing out on the best "heart attack vaccine" modern medicine has to offer.

During a large observational study, researchers from Minneapolis Veterans Affairs Medical Center studied more than 286,000 men and women over age 65 who received flu vaccinations over two flu seasons. They found that compared with people who weren't vaccinated, those who had the shots were 20 percent less likely to be hospitalized for heart disease or stroke, 30 percent less likely to succumb to pneumonia, and half as likely to die from any cause.

In an unrelated study, researchers studying more than 200 men and women with coronary heart disease found that those who got flu shots were 67 percent less likely to have second heart attacks than those who hadn't been vaccinated that year.

Multilayered Protection

Protecting your heart with a shot in the arm may sound like a medical breakthrough, but the suspected link between influenza and heart attacks dates back to the early 1900s, when an excessive number of deaths during the flu epidemics of that time were attributed to heart disease rather than the flu.

Today, researchers speculate that the flu vaccine shields against heart disease by cooling inflammation before it happens. If an invading flu virus can't set up shop and cause infection, your immune system doesn't have to flood your bloodstream with an inflammatory response that can ultimately promote blood clots, damage blood vessel walls, and pave the way for cardiovascular disease and heart attack.

"With this extremely inexpensive and safe intervention, we can keep people out of the hospital, and we can prevent them from dying. There are very few things we can do in medicine that provide these benefits over a very short period of time," says Kristin Nichol, M.D., a lead researcher in the Minneapolis study. "This study definitely establishes a substantial association between the flu and cardiovascular disease."

The government recommends that people with heart disease as well as everyone over the age of 50, young children, and others who are at risk have flu shots each year. Yet many people still bypass this *one simple step* that can protect their hearts and fend off misery-causing infections.

Fight Infection

It stands to reason, say experts, that if inflammation is bad for your arteries, avoiding infections of all kinds is heart smart. Getting a flu shot is one way to do that, but there are more. Here are our favorite quick and easy steps to protect yourself during even the germiest times of year.

Get immunized yearly. The viruses that cause influenza change often, and protection declines within a year of your last shot. Flu season in the United States generally kicks off in December and stretches into April. It takes a week or two for the vaccine to provide protection, so it's best to get your

Flu Shot Notes

A flu vaccine uses inactivated or killed influenza viruses to stimulate your immune system to build up antibodies against the live version. That means a flu shot can't give you the flu, but as with any medical treatment, there is a chance of side effects with a vaccine, although they're very rarely serious. If side effects occur, they usually start soon after the shot and last one to two days. They include:

- Soreness, swelling, or redness at the injection site
- Low-level flu symptoms, such as slight fever, chills, and/or aches
- Headache

People who are allergic to eggs should consult their doctors before getting flu shots, since the vaccine contains small amounts of egg protein. You shouldn't have a shot if you're already sick.

flu shot in the fall. You can also get a pneumococcal vaccine to protect against pneumonia—a good idea if you're over 65 or have heart disease. You can get this one-time immunization (you don't need a booster) at the same time you get your flu shot.

A nasal-spray vaccine, approved in 2003, is good for needlephobics but isn't recommended for young children or adults over 50. Unlike the shot, which contains dead influenza viruses, the nasal vaccine is made with weakened live viruses, so it's less safe for people with reduced immunity.

You can get a flu shot at your doctor's office or from your local health department at various public locations such as malls; or at your workplace.

Wash up. The number one way to decrease your risk of infection is to wash your hands so you don't carry germs into your body when you eat, rub your eyes, or wipe your nose. Don't bother with fancy antibacterial soaps, though; they just contribute to the development of antibiotic-resistant germs. Old-fashioned soap works just as well by loosening germ-laden oil and deposits on the skin so they get swept down the drain when you rinse your hands under running water.

Keep your hands off your face. Try to avoid touching your face with your hands, especially during cold and flu season, when plenty of people around you are bound to be sick and spread the germs on their hands.

Treat high-touch objects. Use disinfectant spray to clean steering wheels, faucets, doorknobs, computer keyboards, and telephones. Wash dishes in hot water and let them dry naturally. In the bathroom, keep toothbrushes and towels separate so they don't touch and use disposable cups rather than a communal rinsing cup.

Eat well and exercise. Eating a healthful diet and getting extra protection with vitamin and mineral supplements can help your body produce a strong army of disease-fighting cells. Getting out of your chair for a daily dose of activity helps circulate those germ-battling cells so they can find—and destroy—invading bacteria and viruses in your bloodstream. Following the 30-Minutes-A-Day Plan will not only help your heart but also boost your immunity.

Moisten your membranes. Indoor heating dries out the protective mucous membranes in your nose and throat, making you more susceptible to infections. When buildings are dry in the winter, use non-medicated saline spray several times a day to clean bacteria and other particles from your nose and keep the membranes moist.

Stop smoking. Smoke damages the tiny hairs in the nose that filter out bacteria and viruses and also depletes essential immunity-building nutrients. That means smokers are far more susceptible to infections, usually have infections that are more severe, and take longer to heal than non-smokers. (See page 192 for advice on quitting smoking.)

A Gum Disease Vaccine for the Heart?

So far, the flu shot is the immunization with the best heart-protection record, but there may be another vaccine on the way that may slash the odds of heart attacks in half for certain high-risk individuals. Researchers at Boston University School of Medicine recently found that they can prevent mice from developing *Porphy-romonas gingivalis*–accelerated heart disease by immunizing them with a vaccine that protects against periodontal disease.

As you learned in the chapter on tooth plaque, chronic bacterial infection of the gums—otherwise known as periodontal disease—can double your risk of having a fatal heart attack. Gum disease, like influenza, creates a state of persistent inflammation that leads to atherosclerosis, or plaque buildup in the arteries. Trials are under way to develop a periodontal vaccine for humans, so ask your dentist to keep you posted. In the meantime, follow the oral hygiene tips on page 200.

Use this hand-drying strategy in public restrooms. Studies find a shockingly large percentage of people fail to wash their hands after using a public restroom. And every single one of them touches the door handle on the way out. So after washing your hands, use a paper towel to turn off the faucet. Use another paper towel to dry your hands, then open the door with that paper towel as a barrier between you and the handle. It sounds nuts, but it's an actual recommendation from the Centers for Disease Control to protect you from infectious diseases like cold and flu.

Carry hand sanitizer with you. Available in gel or towelette forms, these allow you to clean your hands anytime, even if the closest water supply is 100 miles away. And they work. One study of absenteeism due to infection in elementary schools found schools using the gel sanitizer had absentee rates from infection nearly 20 percent lower than those schools using other hand-cleaning methods.

Use your knuckle to rub your eyes. It's less likely to be contaminated with viruses than your fingertip. This is particularly important given that the eye provides a perfect entry point for germs, and the average person rubs his eyes or nose or scratches his face 20-50 times a day.

Put a box of tissues wherever people sit. Come October, buy a 6- or 12-pack of tissue boxes and strategically place them around the house, your workplace, your car. Don't let aesthetics thwart you. You need tissues widely available so that anyone who has to cough or sneeze or blow his nose will do so in the way least likely to spread his germs.

Leave the windows in your house open a crack in winter. Not all of them, but one or two in the rooms in which you spend the most time. This is particularly important if you live in a newer home, where fresh circulating air has been the victim of energy efficiency. A bit of fresh air will do wonders for chasing out germs.

Buy a hygrometer. These little tools measure humidity. You want your home to measure around 50 percent. A consistent measure higher than 60 percent means mold and mildew may start to set in your walls, fabrics, and kitchen; lower than 40 percent and the dry air makes you more susceptible to germs.

Sit in a sauna once a week. Why? Because an Austrian study published in 1990 found that volunteers who frequently used a sauna had half the rate of colds during the six-month study period than those who didn't use a sauna at all. It's possible that the hot air you inhale kills cold viruses. Most gyms have saunas these days.

Take a garlic supplement every day. When 146 volunteers received either one garlic supplement a day or a placebo for 12 weeks between November and February, those taking the garlic were not only less likely to get a cold, but if they did catch one, their symptoms were less intense and they recovered faster.

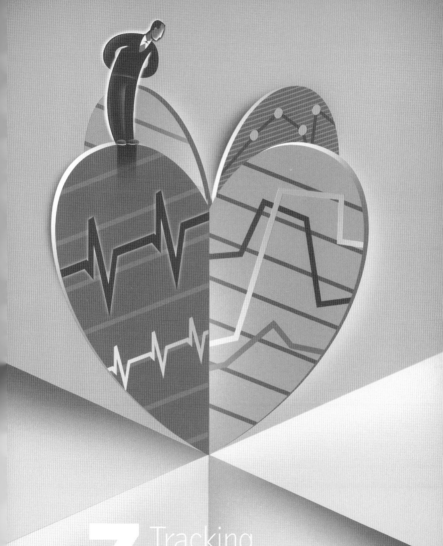

7 Tracking
Well

By tracking just a few numbers and asking yourself a few simple questions, you can have a surprisingly accurate assessment of the health of your heart.

6 Numbers That Can Save Your Life

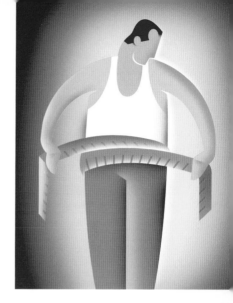

HOW DO YOU MONITOR your financial health? The truth is, there are hundreds of numbers you can track, and if you were a trained expert, you'd follow many of them on an almost daily basis. But for most of us, financial health boils down to just a handful of reliable measurements: our total debt, total assets, monthly income, and the rate of return on investments.

The same holds true for your personal health. There are numerous measurements you could track to the point of obsession, and if you were a doctor, you'd be able to infer meaning from the subtle changes from day to day. For most of us, though, our health status can be revealed by just a few numbers, measured and monitored over time.

Which ones, though?

Ask a hundred doctors, you'll get a hundred different answers.

It seems surprising, but neither the government nor the American Medical Association or any other major health organization has provided guidelines for the best way for individuals to track their health. If pushed, they would tell you to just go to a doctor—he'll know what to track.

Well, we disagree. If each of us is ultimately in charge of our own heart and health, then each of us should know the numbers that best provide a comprehensive report of our physical well-being.

After much consideration, we have chosen six measurements that will do just that—provide a multifaceted view of where you stand in your battle against the six main heart attackers. We believe that every thinking adult should know these important, easy-to-obtain measurements of heart health.

How easy? Three are totally do-it-yourself (all you need is a pencil, a tape measure, and a watch), and the others are standard doctor's-office procedures. Gather these numbers, write them down, and track them over time. Together, they speak volumes about the health of your heart—and your progress on the 30-Minutes-A-Day Plan.

1 DAILY CALORIE NEEDS
Know Your Food Requirements

Okay, this isn't technically a measurement, but it's a number that, if you pay attention to it, can have a huge influence on your health.

How much food should you eat in a day? Back on page 76, we mentioned how few people knew the answer to this question and then gave a basic formula for calculating your calorie needs: from 13 to 15 calories per pound of body weight per day, depending on your activity level.

How much food do you actually eat? Many of us nibble and nosh our way through the day without any real sense of how much we're consuming. In most cases, we are eating much more food than we need.

In a perfect world, the difference between your daily intake and your daily needs would be zero—that is, you'd eat just enough to provide fuel for your body. If you were trying to lose weight safely, you'd eat roughly 500 calories *less* than your body requires. The reality is, though, that many of us eat from 100 to 1,000 calories *more* than we need.

It sounds simple, but no health number is as important—and as instructive—as the one that helps you understand your daily food needs and whether you're exceeding them. The obvious reason is that overeating leads to weight gain, and becoming overweight is among the worst things you can do for your heart and health. The less-than-obvious reason is that eating too many calories usually means eating unhealthy foods, since they're so much higher in calories than natural, healthy foods because of all the fat and sugar in them. It's almost impossible to get too many calories if you focus on eating lots of fruits and vegetables. And having a diet rich in produce means you get loads of vitamins, minerals, antioxidants, and other nutrients essential for heart health.

Most women need approximately 1,800 calories a day for good health. Men typically need about 2,100. That usually equates to 300 to 400 calories for breakfast, 400 to 500 for lunch, 500 to 600 for dinner, and two or three snacks of roughly 100 to 200 calories each.

But don't rely on such broad estimates. Your daily calorie need isn't a static number; it can change over time. If you are exercising more, healing from disease, or in a high-stress period, your body may need extra fuel. If you've lost weight, chances are your body requires less fuel than it once did. Then there's metabolism—some of us burn calories more efficiently than others.

The main message: All adults should have a good understanding of how much food they need to eat each day for optimal health, energy, and weight. The trick is how to do that. Calories are the simplest statistical measure, but steak doesn't have its calorie count stamped on it anywhere, and who wants to look up everything they eat in a calorie counter and keep a tally of it all? The next best way—and the one we recommend—is visual training: learning what, for example, a 300-calorie breakfast looks like. For this kind of help, turn to "Perfect Portion Size Guide" (page 94).

In general, the meals and snacks we mentioned in the 30-Minutes-A-Day Plan add up to 1,500 to 1,800 calories a day. Adjust them as necessary to meet your unique needs.

DAILY CALORIE NEEDS

✓ **How to check:** On this plan, you don't need a calculator and calorie-counting guide to feel confident that you're not overdoing it. We think sticking with the plan's wide range of healthy, recommended foods in the right-size portions is an easier, healthier, and equally accurate way to judge your energy intake.

✓ **How often to check:** For the first two weeks of the plan, check all portions—use our handy guidelines (see page 94) or pull out the measuring cups and spoons to check meals at home. After that, be sure to continue eyeballing portions. One day a week, try to be very conscious of portion sizes at all your meals.

✓ **Why it's important:** It's easy to overeat, and an extra slice of cheese here, an extra helping of meat there, or a soda and a candy bar "just this once" as a snack can add up to unconscious calorie overload. That leads to weight gain, not weight control.

2 WAIST CIRCUMFERENCE
A Top Way to Monitor Body Fat

Surprised? It turns out that of all the ways to measure whether your weight is affecting the health of your heart, waist size is among the best.

Remember that fat cells aren't just storage lockers for extra calories your body can't burn off. When body fat is packed into your abdomen—literally in and around your internal organs—the fat cells act as thousands of dangerous little hormone pumps that churn out inflammatory chemicals and out-of-whack levels of appetite-controlling proteins. The result? Your risk of heart attack soars as inflammation speeds up atherosclerosis. Plus, your risk for insulin resistance and metabolic syndrome rise as inflammatory substances interfere with the way muscle and liver cells function. Meanwhile, your natural appetite-suppressing system is thrown off, leading to even more overeating and more abdominal fat. Unless you have access to sophisticated laboratory scanning equipment that can view fat directly, checking your waist circumference with a tape measure is the best indicator of how much abdominal fat you have inside.

For women, health risk begins to rise with a waist circumference of more than 31 inches; over 35 is a serious threat. For men, risk increases with a measurement of more than 37, with over 40 being serious.

WAIST CIRCUMFERENCE

✓ **How to check:** Wrap a tape measure around your body in the middle of your abdomen, at or near your belly button. Keep it snug but not tight—and don't suck in your gut. (No one else has to know your number!)

✓ **How often to check:** Every two weeks. (A note for women: Try not to measure in the week before and during your menstrual period, when water retention may bloat your belly and give a false measurement.)

✓ **Why it's important:** Regular checks will help you track your progress as belly fat melts away on the 30-Minutes-A-Day Plan. It will also remind you to get back on the program if you slip off.

3 LDLS AND HDLS
Cholesterol Counts *Do* Count

We've "cheated" here and included two numbers in one category—for two good reasons. First, it's important to know not just how high or low your "bad" LDL cholesterol levels are but also whether your "good" HDLs are up to the challenge of mopping up extra LDLs to protect your arteries. Second, we want to be certain you ask for and receive a detailed cholesterol report each time your doctor checks your blood lipids. Knowing only your total cholesterol won't give you the specifics you and your doctor need to accurately assess and reverse heart risk.

We recommend that you strive for LDLs below 100 mg/dl, especially if you have a history of heart attack or known heart disease. Levels up to 130 are considered nearly optimal; above 130 is high. For women, healthy HDLs should be 50 to 60 mg/dl or higher; for men, their HDLs should be 40 to 50 mg/dl and above.

LDLS AND HDLS

✓ **How to check:** Your doctor will check your cholesterol after you've fasted for 8 to 12 hours. We recommend doctor's-office checks instead of home cholesterol test kits, which are usually less accurate and can't give you those all-important LDL and HDL numbers.

✓ **How often to check:** Once a year if your LDLs and HDLs are within healthy ranges or as often as every three months if your cholesterol is high and you're working actively to lower it.

✓ **Why it's important:** LDL and HDL levels are among the strongest predictors of heart attack risk. Regular checkups will help you notice trends (Are your LDLs steadily rising? Your HDLs slowly falling?) and give you a chance to take steps to correct problems before they happen.

4 BLOOD PRESSURE
An Indicator of Artery Health

Blood pressure—the force of blood against the walls of your arteries—rises and falls naturally during the day. When it remains elevated, you have hypertension and with it, a higher risk of atherosclerosis, heart disease, and stroke.

A reading of 140/90 mm/Hg or more is considered high, but if it's between 120/80 and 139/89, you have prehypertension and should take steps to prevent the development of hypertension. The movement program and eating plan in this book—full of fruits, veggies, and low-fat dairy products—can help.

BLOOD PRESSURE

✓ **How to check:** If your pressure is normal, the standard advice is have a retest every two years. But a new study published in the *Journal of the American Medical Association* found that 13 percent of people whose pressure seemed normal in the doctor's office actually turned out to have high blood pressure when they checked at home. We suggest talking with your doctor about the pros and cons of getting a home blood pressure monitor (she can help you figure out which type is best for you) and getting instructions on how to use it.

✓ **How often to check:** If your doctor doesn't recommend a home test, ask for a blood pressure check at every doctor's visit. Also take advantage of other opportunities to check it—at community blood pressure checks, workplace health fairs, and even blood pressure testing machines at the drugstore. These aren't substitutes for doctor's-office checks, but they'll help you track your personal BP trends.

✓ **Why it's important:** Regular checks will help spot a potential problem early, when lifestyle changes are more likely to resolve high blood pressure.

5 TRIGLYCERIDES
The *Other* Type of Fat to Watch

Triglycerides are chemical packages that contain extra calories your cells can't burn right after a meal. They're made from the carbs and fats you eat, which are converted into a form that can be stored in fat cells. Triglycerides are also released from fat tissue when the body needs extra energy between meals. It's normal to have some triglycerides in your bloodstream, but extra-high levels are linked to coronary artery disease, especially in women. When you have high triglycerides paired with low HDLs, your risk of insulin resistance and metabolic syndrome may be elevated.

A normal triglyceride reading is less than 150 mg/dl. Borderline high levels are 150 to 199 mg/dl, and over 200 is high.

TRIGLYCERIDES

✓ **How to check:** A triglyceride check is usually done with the same blood sample your doctor draws for a fasting cholesterol test.

✓ **How often to check:** Test triglycerides once a year if your levels are normal or as often as every three months if they're high.

✓ **Why it's important:** Regular checks are an important early warning system for your heart.

6 MORNING PULSE RATE
Know If Your Heart Is Strong

Your pulse is the number of times your heart beats in 1 minute. Regular monitoring of your resting pulse, first thing in the morning, will help you see if your exercise program is strengthening your heart. It will also help you spot problems that can't be found with the other checks mentioned in this chapter.

For example, a normal resting pulse rate is 60 to 90 beats per minute. Normally, people in better physical condition have lower resting rates because their heart muscles are in good shape, and each beat is strong and forceful. If you're not a regular exerciser and your heart rate is lower than the normal range, tell your doctor—it could be a sign of heart disease. When checking your pulse, also notice how the beats feel. A healthy pulse feels soft yet firm against your fingers; a weak pulse feels faint and could indicate heart failure. If your pulse feels hard and pounding, it could be a sign of atherosclerosis, and an irregular rhythm could be a sign of a heart abnormality. Tell your doc if you notice anything unusual about the "feel" of your pulse.

MORNING PULSE RATE

✓ **How to check:** You'll need a clock or watch with a second hand. The pulse is best measured at the wrist or neck, where an artery runs close to the surface of the skin. To measure the pulse at your wrist, place your index and middle fingers on the underside of the opposite wrist. Press firmly with the flat of your fingers until you feel the pulse. For a neck measurement, gently press your index and middle fingers against your neck in the hollow just below and in front of the back corner of your jawbone.

After you've found your pulse, count the beats for 1 minute (or count for 30 seconds and multiply by two). The result is your pulse rate in beats per minute.

✓ **How often to check:** Take your pulse once a month, before you get out of bed in the morning.

✓ **Why it's important:** This check has two purposes. It will show you whether your exercise program is strengthening your heart (if your pulse rate gradually falls within the healthy range). It will also give you a heads-up about a variety of heart problems.

Your Health— By the Numbers

Using your doctor and this book for guidance, determine your current measurements and set reasonable targets. Then check off the actions you're willing to take to achieve your goals.

DAILY CALORIE NEEDS

Estimated daily calories: _____
Target daily calories: _____
Calorie surplus: _____

Actions to improve
- ___ Eat fewer snacks
- ___ Cut back on fatty foods
- ___ Eat more vegetables and fruit
- ___ Have one no-meat meal each day

WAIST CIRCUMFERENCE

Current waist size: _____
Target waist size: _____

Actions to improve
- ___ Cut back on daily calories
- ___ Take brisk daily walks
- ___ Maintain a strength-building program
- ___ Maintain a stretching program

LDLS AND HDLS

Current HDLs: _____
Target HDLs: _____
Current LDLs: _____
Target LDLs: _____

Actions to improve
- ___ Increase daily fiber intake
- ___ Eat more fish, olive oil, and nuts
- ___ Get sterols daily from capsules or margarine
- ___ Exercise regularly
- ___ Consider a niacin supplement

BLOOD PRESSURE

Current blood pressure: _____
Target blood pressure: _____

Actions to improve
- ___ Cut way back on salt
- ___ Take a daily multivitamin
- ___ Consider a daily coenzyme Q_{10} supplement
- ___ Eat high-calcium foods

TRIGLYCERIDES

Current triglycerides: _____
Target triglycerides: _____

Actions to improve
- ___ Replace simple carbs with complex carbs
- ___ Drink only in moderation
- ___ Eat more vegetables every day
- ___ Cut back on saturated fats
- ___ Consider a fish-oil supplement

MORNING PULSE RATE

Current rate: _____
Target rate: _____

Actions to improve
- ___ Get heart-pumping exercise regularly
- ___ Learn relaxation techniques to lower stress
- ___ Get a full night's sleep every night
- ___ Lose excess weight

4 Numbers to Track Every Day

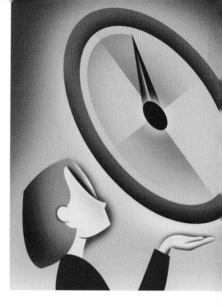

IN THIS BOOK, you've discovered literally hundreds of new ways to fit naturally nutritious foods, heart-protecting supplements, physical activity, and relaxation into your day. Each time you choose one of these strategies, you're taking a step toward a healthier lifestyle. But old habits die hard, and the roadside is filled with alluring, unhealthy diversions. It's easy to order the large fries, watch a Seinfeld re-run instead of turning in at 10 p.m., or choose the 12-inch hoagie and eat the whole thing.

How will you know that you've adopted enough new, healthy habits to make a difference? Easy—just use our simple, daily tracking system.

Here's how it works: Each evening, take just one minute to ask yourself four questions about your day. These four questions distill the key messages and advice of the 30-Minutes-A-Day Plan down to their essence. They won't change, ever, so remembering what they are is a cinch.

Your answers will make it instantly apparent whether you a staying true to the path toward health, or if your good intentions are not being matched with good actions.

If you find the latter to be the case more often than not, ask yourself these four questions in the late afternoon instead of the evening. By doing so, you'll give yourself plenty of time to make healthy choices come dinner and evening time.

Remember: to travel easily on the road to a long, healthy life, you want your steps to be natural and painless. A daily check-in makes sure you are traveling just that way. Here are the details:

1 FRUIT AND VEGETABLE CONSUMPTION

If you make just one change because of the 30-Minutes-A-Day Plan, let it be adding produce to every meal you eat. Fruits and veggies lower heart disease by pumping your body full of soluble and insoluble fiber, flooding your bloodstream and cells with artery-protecting antioxidants, and delivering vitamins and minerals that help control blood pressure and keep arteries flexible.

FRUIT AND VEGETABLE CONSUMPTION

✓ **Ask yourself:** Did I have nine produce servings today?

✓ **Your goal:** Four fruit servings and five vegetable servings

✓ **Tracking trick:** For women: Wear nine bangle bracelets on the same arm. Each time you have a fruit or veggie, move one bracelet to the other arm. For men: Keep nine paperclips in your pants pocket. Move one to another pocket for each serving of produce you consume.

✓ **Extra credit:** Aim to put a riot of color on your plate every day—green broccoli, purple grapes, yellow squash, red tomatoes, and orange peaches, for example.

✓ **How to catch up:** If you've had breakfast and lunch with little or no produce, make up lost ground with a fruit snack in the afternoon, a big salad for dinner, and another fruit snack in the evening.

2 FIBER CONSUMPTION

Fiber at every meal keeps blood sugar from spiking. This controls cravings, helps you feel full and stay full longer, and lowers diabetes and heart disease risk. But the benefits don't stop there: Getting soluble fiber (from oatmeal, barley, or a supplement) slashes cholesterol levels. High-fiber foods are also less processed, so you get a whole package of naturally balanced, heart-pampering nutrients at the same time. Whole grains also provide vitamin E and other antioxidants. High-fiber nuts give you good fats—monounsaturated fat to preserve "good" HDLs and, if you choose walnuts, omega-3s to keep your heart beating at a steady rhythm.

FIBER CONSUMPTION

✓ **Ask yourself:** Did I have three whole grains plus some nuts and/or beans today?

✓ **Your goal:** Two to four servings of whole grains and one or two servings of nuts and/or beans

✓ **Tracking trick:** Think 3-2-1. That's three whole grains, two fiber supplements, and one serving of nuts.

✓ **Extra credit:** Make at least one of your fiber-rich grains a soluble-fiber powerhouse such as oatmeal or barley; take one or two soluble-fiber supplements.

✓ **How to catch up:** Had a low-fiber breakfast and lunch? Snack on nuts this afternoon and have beans in your main dish at dinner—in chili, a burrito, or as a quick salad topper—with a slice of whole wheat bread.

3 RELAXATION TIME

Consciously relaxing doesn't mean taking an hour out of your busy day to meditate or have a massage (although if you can do either, you'll feel great!). There are dozens of ways to relax without stopping what you're doing: You can practice mindfulness—being fully present and aware of what you're doing—or take a few minutes to focus on your breathing. You can let go of impatient thoughts before they double your risk of high blood pressure and heart attack. And don't underestimate the soothing health benefits of sharing a laugh with friends, listening to music, walking and petting your dog, or enjoying nature.

RELAXATION TIME

✓ **Ask yourself:** Did I take at least 15 minutes to de-stress today?

✓ **Your goal:** Get that relaxed feeling every day.

✓ **Tracking trick:** Check in with yourself several times a day. You'll know if you're stressed.

✓ **Extra credit:** Once a week, try to spend an hour immersed in something you love—gardening, a sport, reading, or whatever else gives you pleasure.

✓ **How to catch up:** In the midst of a stressed-out day, remind yourself that you'll be more productive if you take a few minutes to breathe deeply and unwind.

Surprising Signs of Success

You don't need a medical degree and a stethoscope to see that your efforts are paying off. Long before you go back to your doctor for a blood pressure check and a new cholesterol test, the following lifestyle measurements of success will show you that you're on the right track. Expect to begin experiencing these benefits fast—some within a week or two of starting this plan.

• **More energy.** You've got more vim and vigor all day, even during the 3 p.m. slump.

• **Better sleep.** Your slumber is deeper; you wake up feeling more refreshed.

• **A tighter belt.** You can take it in an extra notch or two.

• **Better-fitting clothes.** You look better in your pants or skirts, and you can wear your "skinny jeans" again!

• **More money in your wallet.** You've got cash left over from the food budget at week's end because you're eating less fast food and buying fewer processed items.

• **Better moods.** Little annoyances roll right off your back, and you're laughing more. Your outlook is more optimistic.

• **More strength.** It's easier to lift the grocery bags or pick up your kids or grandkids.

• **Real muscles.** Are those biceps rippling in your upper arms? Your muscles are gaining definition. Nice.

4 MOVEMENT TIME

Physical activity controls weight, burns off belly fat, lowers high blood pressure, and tames out-of-line cholesterol levels. It even cools inflammation and helps your cells absorb more blood sugar, cutting the risk of type 2 diabetes. On the 30-Minutes-A-Day Plan, you've discovered dozens of ways to build activity into your daily life—plus a simple plan for strength training to build muscle density and walking to boost cardiovascular fitness.

MOVEMENT TIME

✓ **Ask yourself:** Did I get on my feet for fun or exercise today?

✓ **Your goal:** Sit for 1 hour less per day. Fit in a morning toning routine and a brisk, short stroll or two during the day.

✓ **Tracking trick:** Before lunch and at midafternoon, ask yourself how long you've been sitting without a break. Chances are, it's time to get up and move.

✓ **Extra credit:** Build short bursts of intensity into your daily movement routine—pump your arms and stride quickly up a hill or walk in place briskly while you're chatting on the phone.

✓ **How to catch up:** At the end of a day that left you no time to leave your chair, be sure to take the stairs, not the elevator. Stroll around outside for a few minutes before getting into your car. Once at home, take the dog for a walk and drag the kids out for a game of Frisbee or tag. At night, use commercial breaks during your favorite TV show to do the exercises on page 154.

Do I Get a Day Off?

Short answer: No.

Longer, more compassionate answer: If you are feeling pressured by your new health regimen, and are seeking a "day off" from "being good," then you need to be reminded of the fundamental truth about healthy living. And that is: It's not a program that you can go on or off of. It's not a formal diet, or rigid exercise regimen, or mandatory stress-relief program, or a weekly visit to the psychiatrist, doctor, nutritionist, trainer, or salon.

Health is about how you live, each and every moment. It's about sleeping well, and waking up happy, and eating a good breakfast, and enjoying your work, and taking regular breaks, and laughing with friend and family, and having a good attitude, and enjoying fresh foods, and loving nature, and respecting yourself. Not just some of the time, but almost all of the time. It's the difference between the regular day and the heart-healthy day we described back on page 46.

Look at it this way: you are going to sleep, work, eat, have leisure time each and every day. Health is achieved by going about these activities a little smarter, a little healthier, with a slightly different attitude. As we've said, it's the little choices that matter: whole wheat toast, not white toast; a walk, not a sitcom; laughter, not anger. These types of every-moment choices are what cleans arteries, lowers blood pressure, strengthens the heart, and makes life long and good. Along the way, a little ice cream, an occasional steak, a lethargic afternoon doesn't really matter, because it is more than balanced out with your everyday good choices.

So if you still believe health is achieved by doing a program, it's time to break free. Yes, a formal program can get you started, teach you healthy choices, help you break bad habits and form better ones. And in fact, that's what the following section is all about. But in the end, healthy living, done right, is merely living. But such a good kind of living.

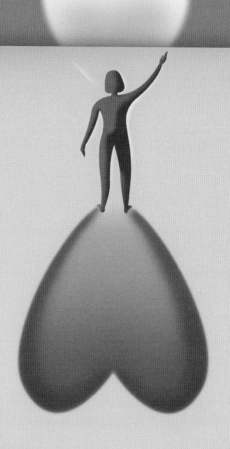

8 The 30-Minutes-A-Day
Plan Workbook

The reward of healthy living is not merely
a healthy heart sometime in the
future. Healthy living is
like the sun—warming,
invigorating, and uplifting,
all *the time.*

Putting the Healthy Heart Plan to Work

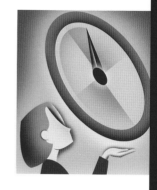

As we've said, the 30-Minutes-A-Day Plan is not a rigid program. Instead, our plan is a promise—that it will take no more than 30 minutes each day to integrate the small changes into your life that will deliver you a strong, well-protected heart. But what exactly do you do once you put this book down?

The following pages are dedicated to answering that. Our goal is to make it as easy as possible to embark—and succeed—on the 30-Minutes-A-Day Plan. Here is what you'll find:

The Healthy Heart Starter Kit: You've made the commitment; now it's time to take action. Refer back to the "Getting Started" chapter on page 48 for guidance on your unique priorities. Then turn to this checklist to commit to the specific changes you want to do: first, second, and third.

Use these guidelines to prioritize your goals and to determine how much you can reasonably change (remember, a heart-healthy lifestyle is sustainable!). Whether you would like to modify your eating habits, incorporate more activity into your life, or simply reduce everyday stress through spirituality or by spending more quality time with your family, the first step to success is defining your goals.

Healthy Heart Recipes: Here are 41 fresh, chef-tested recipes, all developed as much for taste as for healthiness with less than 30 percent of calories from fat and using natural, healthy ingredients. Be good to your heart and your stomach with delicious, filling and nutritious entrées like Lemony Salmon Patties (page 236) and Beef and Turkey Chili (page 240). Trying to include your family in your healthy new lifestyle? Your spouse and children won't complain when you serve up classic dishes like New England Clam Chowder (page 229) and Oven Fries (page 232)—and they're good for you too! You don't have to banish your sweet tooth; just check out our dessert recipes—delicious treats that will have your heart beating better than ever.

The Healthy Heart Starter Kit

The secret to success with the 30-Minutes-A-Day Plan is to slowly, steadily exchange unhealthy habits and practices with heart-healthy ones. So review the following list of suggested changes, and mark appropriate ones as follows:

I: Immediate—I want to start this immediately!
N: Next—Once I integrate the first round of changes into my life, I intend to tackle this.
C: Committed—This is not an immediate priority, but I'll make this happen in the months ahead.
R: Research—I want to know more about this before committing and will reread about it in this book and do additional investigating.

EATING

__ Eat a healthier breakfast

__ Eat a healthier lunch

__ Eat a healthier dinner

__ Commit to more vegetables at my meals

__ Switch to healthier carbs (whole grain bread, brown rice, sweet potatoes)

__ Eat more seafood

__ Eat healthier, less-processed snacks

__ Reduce my intake of corn syrup and sugar

__ Drink more water

__ Drink less soda

__ Eat less junk food (chips, candy, ice cream, cookies)

__ Stop eating out of habit, boredom, or stress

__ Plan my dinners in advance

__ Shop from a shopping list

__ Eat less from fast-food restaurants

__ (Other) _____
_____

MOVING

__ Start each morning with a stretching routine

__ Do five minutes of strength exercises a day

__ Take a long, vigorous walk every day

__ Sneak in more short walks throughout the day

__ Commit to being on my feet more throughout the day

__ Give yoga a try

__ Resume or start an active hobby like gardening, rowing, or biking

__ (Other) _____
_____

LIVING

__ Work at getting angry less often

__ Work at managing stress more effectively

__ Find ways to laugh more

__ Be more forgiving of myself and others

__ Be more loving to friends and family

__ Reinvigorate my spirituality and recommit to a higher purpose in life

__ Lose a destructive habit, such as smoking or excessive drinking

__ Get more sleep each night

__ Commit to a daily multivitamin

__ Commit to other heart-healthy supplements

__ Switch to less toxic cleaning methods

__ Commence a more thorough daily mouth-care regimen that includes flossing

__ Wash hands more frequently and be more diligent in blocking germs

__ Answer the four essential health questions each evening (detailed on page 218-220):

__ (Other) _____
_____

Which changes do you plan to start immediately? *(If you picked more than five, go back over your list and change several to "N," or "next." Overcommitting is the wrong path to success. Start simply, and succeed!)*

1. _____
2. _____
3. _____
4. _____
5. _____

What must you buy to get started? _____
_____
_____

How must you adjust your schedule to get started?_____
_____
_____

How will you reward yourself for successes?
In three days_____
In a week_____
In a month_____

What is your next set of changes?

1. _____
2. _____
3. _____
4. _____
5. _____

How will you trigger yourself to embark on these new changes? *(Suggestions include scheduling them on your calendar, using the start of each month or the arrival of a monthly magazine as a reassessment, asking a loved one to remind you, using holidays or the seasons to trigger some new goals)*
_____
_____
_____

What are your three-month goals?_____
_____

How will you reward yourself for full success?_____
_____

How will you reward yourself for partial success?_____
_____

How will you remotivate yourself if only limited success?_____
_____

Healthy Heart Recipes

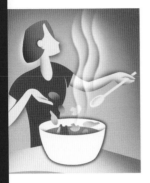

There are lots of cookbooks that claim to offer recipes that are "healthy" but never bother to define the term. In fairness, that's partly because there is no formal definition of a healthy recipe, and one doctor's opinion often conflicts with another's.

Well, we're stating our definition here and now. The following are the criteria for dishes that we consider truly heart healthy; they're the ones we used to develop the recipes in the pages ahead. Our recipes:

- Use a minimal number of processed foods
- Feature mostly fresh ingredients, particularly vegetables or fruits
- Use whole, unrefined carbohydrates
- Use a minimal amount of refined sugar
- Have less than 800 milligrams of sodium per serving
- Have less than 30 percent of calories from fat
- Have less than 10 percent of calories from saturated fat
- For entrées, have less than 600 calories per serving
- For snacks/side dishes, have less than 150 calories per serving
- Use proven heart-healthy ingredients, such as salmon, flaxseed oil, olive oil, canola oil, avocados, cocoa, soy, beans, garlic, turmeric, ginger, cinnamon, cumin, and cholesterol-lowering margarine (such as Benecol or Take Control)

Did we allow a few exceptions? Sure. Sometimes using a healthy fat like olive oil can push the fat calories over 30 percent. If the dish is otherwise healthy, that's a fair exception to the rule. Similarly, a fruity, nutty dessert may exceed 150 calories, but if it's made with all healthy ingredients, then it's okay to splurge occasionally. Just don't make exceptions more than a few times a week.

Now, we know that most people don't eat meals that are anywhere close to these healthy standards. Don't despair! Take it one small step at time. Start by reducing portion sizes, then add a few more fruits and vegetables. Next, work to break your butter habit. With time and practice, you'll discover that you're naturally choosing the healthy alternative—and that your weight is dropping and your health improving.

▶ Corn Salsa Tostadas

Makes 3 dozen

3 flour tortillas (8 inches)

$^3/_4$ cup fat-free sour cream

2 scallions, finely chopped

$^1/_4$ teaspoon garlic powder

3 teaspoons minced cilantro or parsley

$^3/_4$ cup fresh or thawed frozen corn

1 plum tomato, finely chopped

1 tablespoon chopped jalapeño pepper*

2 tablespoons orange juice

1 teaspoon canola oil

$^1/_2$ teaspoon salt

1. Using a 2-inch-round cookie cutter, cut 12 circles from each tortilla. Coat both sides of the circles with cooking spray. Place in a single layer on a baking sheet and bake at 400°F until crisp, 4 to 5 minutes. Set aside to cool.

2. In a small bowl, combine the sour cream, scallions, garlic powder, and 1 teaspoon cilantro. Cover and refrigerate.

3. In a medium bowl, combine the corn, tomato, jalapeño, orange juice, oil, salt, and the remaining cilantro. Cover and refrigerate. Just before serving, spread 1 teaspoon of the sour cream mixture over each tostada. Using a slotted spoon, top each with a teaspoon of salsa.

*Editor's Note: When cutting or seeding hot peppers, use rubber or plastic gloves to protect your hands. Avoid touching your face.

Per serving *(6 tostadas): 141 calories, 3 g fat, 0 g saturated fat, 3 mg cholesterol, 347 mg sodium, 25 g carbohydrate, 1 g fiber, 5 g protein.*

▶ Vegetable Spiral Sticks

Makes 2 dozen

3 medium carrots

12 spears fresh asparagus, trimmed

$^1/_4$ cup grated Parmesan cheese

$^1/_2$ teaspoon dried oregano

1 tube (11 ounces) refrigerated breadstick dough

1 egg white, beaten

1. Cut the carrots lengthwise into quarters. In a large skillet, bring 2 inches of water to a boil. Add the carrots and cook 3 minutes. Add the asparagus and cook 2 to 3 minutes longer. Drain, rinse with cold water, and pat dry.

2. Preheat the oven to 375°F. Coat a baking sheet with cooking spray. In a small bowl, combine the Parmesan and oregano.

3. Cut each piece of breadstick dough in half and roll into a 7-inch rope. Wrap one rope in a spiral around each vegetable. Place on the baking sheet and tuck the ends of the dough under the vegetables to secure. Brush with the egg white. Sprinkle the cheese mixture over the sticks and bake until golden brown, 7 to 14 minutes. Serve warm.

Per serving *(2 sticks): 97 calories, 2 g fat, 0 g saturated fat, 2 mg cholesterol, 247 mg sodium, 15 g carbohydrate, 1 g fiber, 4 g protein.*

▶ Savory Potato Skins

Makes 32 shells

4 large baking potatoes, baked

1 teaspoon garlic powder

1 teaspoon paprika

1 teaspoon salt *(optional)*

Fat-free sour cream *(optional)*

Chives *(optional)*

1. Preheat the broiler. Coat a baking sheet with cooking spray.

2. Cut the potatoes in half lengthwise and scoop out the pulp, leaving a 1/4-inch-thick shell. (Save the pulp for another use.) Cut the shells lengthwise into quarters, place on the baking sheet, and mist with cooking spray.

3. In a small bowl, combine the garlic powder, paprika, and salt (if desired). Sprinkle over the skins. Broil until golden brown, 5 to 8 minutes. If desired, combine the sour cream and chives and serve with the potato skins.

Per serving *(4 shells, calculated without salt and sour cream and chives): 70 calories, 0 g fat, 0 g saturated fat, 0 mg cholesterol, 5 mg sodium, 17 g carbohydrate, 1 g fiber, 2 g protein.*

▶ Cinnamon Popcorn

Makes 8 servings

8 cups plain popped popcorn

1 egg white, lightly beaten

1/2 cup sugar

1 teaspoon ground cinnamon

1/4 teaspoon salt *(optional)*

1. Preheat the oven to 300°F. Place the popcorn in a 15 x 10 x 1-inch baking pan.

2. In a small bowl, combine the egg white, sugar, cinnamon, and salt (if desired). Pour over the popcorn and mix well. Bake for 20 minutes. Let cool and store in an airtight container.

Per serving *(1 cup, calculated without salt): 91 calories, 1 g fat, 0 g saturated fat, 0 mg cholesterol, 7 mg sodium, 21 g carbohydrate, 2 g fiber, 3 g protein.*

▶ Oatmeal Waffles

Makes 8 waffles (4 inches) or 16 pancakes

½ cup liquid egg substitute
2 cups buttermilk
1 cup quick-cooking oats
1 tablespoon molasses
1 tablespoon vegetable oil
1 cup whole wheat flour
½ teaspoon salt
1 teaspoon baking soda
1 teaspoon baking powder
  Confectioners' sugar
  Fresh strawberries
  (optional)

1. Coat a waffle maker or pancake griddle with cooking spray. Preheat the waffle maker or griddle.

2. In a large bowl, combine the egg substitute and buttermilk. Add the oats and mix well. Stir in the molasses and oil.

3. In a medium bowl, combine the flour, salt, baking soda, and baking powder. Stir into the egg mixture.

4. For waffles, pour the batter onto the waffle maker and bake according to the manufacturer's directions. For pancakes, drop the batter by about ¼ cupfuls onto the griddle and turn when bubbles begin to form on top. If desired, dust with confectioners' sugar and top with strawberries.

Per serving *(1 waffle or 2 pancakes, calculated without confectioners' sugar and strawberries): 160 calories, 4 g fat, 1 g saturated fat, 5 mg cholesterol, 430 mg sodium, 25 g carbohydrate, 3 g fiber, 8 g protein.*

▶ Hearty Ham Scramble

Makes 6 servings

⅓ cup chopped onion
¼ cup chopped green bell pepper
2 medium potatoes, peeled, cooked, and cubed
1½ cups cubed cooked low-fat ham
1½ cups liquid egg substitute
2 tablespoons water
  Dash fresh-ground black pepper

1. Coat a large skillet with cooking spray. Add the onion and bell pepper and cook until crisp-tender. Add the potatoes and ham and cook, stirring, for 5 minutes.

2. In a medium bowl, combine the egg substitute, water, and pepper. Pour over the ham mixture and cook over low heat, stirring occasionally, until the eggs are completely set.

Per serving: *141 calories, 4 g fat, 1 g saturated fat, 17 mg cholesterol, 614 mg sodium, 11 g carbohydrate, 1 g fiber, 15 g protein.*

▶ Apple-Topped Oatcakes

Makes 8 servings

Oatcakes

1½ cups fat-free milk
¾ cup old-fashioned oats
1 egg
1 tablespoon vegetable oil
2 tablespoons molasses
1 cup all-purpose flour
1½ teaspoons baking powder
¾ teaspoon ground cinnamon
¼ teaspoon ground ginger
¼ teaspoon baking soda
¼ teaspoon salt
3 egg whites

Lemon Apples

1 tablespoon margarine
5 medium tart apples, peeled and sliced
1 tablespoon lemon juice
1 teaspoon grated lemon zest
½ cup sugar
1 tablespoon cornstarch
⅛ teaspoon ground nutmeg

1. *To make the oatcakes:* Heat the milk in a medium saucepan. In a large bowl, combine the milk and oats and let stand for 5 minutes. Stir in the egg, oil, and molasses. In a medium bowl, combine the flour, baking powder, cinnamon, ginger, baking soda, and salt. Stir into the oat mixture just until moistened. In a small bowl, beat the egg whites until soft peaks form, then gently fold into the batter. Set aside.

2. Coat a griddle with cooking spray. Preheat the griddle.

3. *To make the lemon apples:* Heat the margarine in a large skillet until foamy. Add the apples, lemon juice, and lemon zest. Cook, stirring occasionally, for 8 to 10 minutes.

4. Meanwhile, pour the oatcake batter by ¼ cupfuls onto the griddle. Cook until bubbles form, then turn and cook until browned.

5. In a small bowl, combine the sugar, cornstarch, and nutmeg. Add to the apple mixture and cook until tender, 2 minutes longer. Serve warm over the oatcakes.

Per serving: *264 calories, 5 g fat, 1 g saturated fat, 28 mg cholesterol, 261 mg sodium, 50 g carbohydrate, 3 g fiber, 7 g protein.*

▶ Potatoes O'Brien

Makes 4 servings

1 tablespoon vegetable oil
¹⁄₂ cup chopped onion
¹⁄₂ cup chopped green bell pepper
¹⁄₂ cup chopped red bell pepper
4 medium red potatoes, cubed
¹⁄₄ cup low-sodium beef stock
¹⁄₂ teaspoon Worcestershire sauce

1. Heat the oil in a large skillet over medium heat. Add the onion, peppers, and potatoes and cook 4 minutes.

2. In a small bowl, combine the stock and Worcestershire sauce, then pour over the vegetables. Cover and cook, stirring occasionally, until the potatoes are tender, 10 minutes. Uncover and cook until the liquid is absorbed, about 3 minutes.

Per serving: 134 calories, 4 g fat, 0 g saturated fat, 0 mg cholesterol, 20 mg sodium, 23 g carbohydrate, 3 g fiber, 3 g protein.

▶ Hearty Carrot Muffins

Makes 1 dozen

³⁄₄ cup fat-free milk
¹⁄₂ cup maple syrup
2 egg whites
1 tablespoon canola oil
¹⁄₂ cup grated tart apple
¹⁄₂ cup shredded carrot
³⁄₄ cup whole wheat flour
¹⁄₂ cup wheat bran
¹⁄₄ cup all-purpose flour
3 tablespoons sugar
1 teaspoon baking powder
1 teaspoon baking soda
¹⁄₂ teaspoon salt
¹⁄₂ teaspoon ground cinnamon

1. Coat a 12-cup muffin pan with cooking spray. Preheat the oven to 375°F.

2. In a large bowl, beat the milk, syrup, egg whites, and oil until smooth. Stir in the apple and carrot. In a small bowl, combine the wheat flour, bran, all-purpose flour, sugar, baking powder, baking soda, salt, and cinnamon. Stir into the milk mixture just until moistened.

3. Fill the muffin cups two-thirds full. Bake until a toothpick inserted in the center of a muffin comes out clean, 18 to 20 minutes. Let the muffins cool in the pan for 5 minutes, then remove and place on a wire rack.

Per serving (1 muffin): 109 calories, 1 g fat, 0 g saturated fat, 0 mg cholesterol, 242 mg sodium, 23 g carbohydrate, 2 g fiber, 3 g protein.

▶ Cream of Leek and Potato Soup

Makes 7½ cups

1 tablespoon olive or canola oil

8 ounces leeks, thickly sliced (white parts only)

1 large onion, coarsely chopped

6 cups chicken or vegetable stock

1 pound all-purpose potatoes, peeled and chopped

⅛ teaspoon salt

⅛ teaspoon ground white pepper

⅓ cup low-fat sour cream

Chopped chives *(optional)*

1. Heat the oil in a 4-quart saucepan over medium heat. Stir in the leeks and onion, then add ¾ cup of the stock. Cover and cook, stirring frequently, until soft but not browned, about 10 minutes.

2. Add the potatoes and stir to coat with the leek mixture. Pour in half of the remaining stock and bring to a boil. Simmer, partially covered, until the potatoes are very soft, 15 to 20 minutes. Remove from the heat and ladle the vegetables and broth into a blender or food processor. Puree until very smooth.

3. Pour the remaining stock into the pan. Add the vegetable puree and simmer, stirring constantly, for 2 to 3 minutes. Add the salt and pepper, then remove from the heat and stir in the sour cream. Ladle into soup bowls and top with the chives (if desired).

Per serving *(1 cup): 111 calories, 3 g fat, 1 g saturated fat, 2 mg cholesterol, 105 mg sodium, 17 g carbohydrate, 2 g fiber, 4 g protein.*

▶ Turkey Tomato Soup

Makes 12 cups

4 pounds tomatoes, seeded and chopped (about 8 large)

3 medium green bell peppers, chopped

2 cans (14½ ounces each) reduced-sodium chicken stock

1 can (14½ ounces) vegetable stock

1½ cups water

1½ teaspoons beef bouillon granules

2 cloves garlic, minced

1 teaspoon dried oregano

1 teaspoon dried basil

½ teaspoon fresh-ground black pepper

3 cups cubed cooked turkey breast

3 cups cooked elbow macaroni

Minced fresh basil *(optional)*

In a large saucepan or Dutch oven, combine the tomatoes, peppers, chicken and vegetable stock, water, bouillon, garlic, oregano, basil, and pepper. Bring to a boil, then reduce the heat, cover, and simmer for 2 hours. Stir in the turkey and macaroni and heat through. Sprinkle with the basil (if desired).

Per serving *(1 cup): 150 calories, 3 g fat, 1 g saturated fat, 28 mg cholesterol, 221 mg sodium, 17 g carbohydrate, 2 g fiber, 14 g protein.*

▶ New England Clam Chowder

Makes 8½ cups

1 dozen littleneck or cherrystone clams or 1 can (10 ounces) whole baby clams, drained and rinsed

6 cups fish stock

1 ounce lean salt pork or reduced-sodium bacon, coarsely chopped

2 large onions, coarsely chopped

1 pound all-purpose potatoes, peeled and chopped

2 cups 1% milk

⅛ teaspoon salt

⅛ teaspoon fresh-ground black pepper

2 tablespoons chopped parsley

1. If using fresh clams, cook in a large saucepan in ¼ cup of the stock. Let cool, then remove from the shells. Coarsely shop either fresh or canned clams and set aside.

2. Cook the pork in a 4-quart saucepan over medium heat until crisp and fat is rendered, about 3 minutes. With a slotted spoon, remove the pork and discard. (If using bacon, reserve for garnish.)

3. Add the onions and ¼ cup of the stock to the pan. Sauté until softened but not browned, about 5 minutes. Stir in the potatoes and remaining stock and bring to a boil. Reduce the heat and partially cover, then simmer, stirring occasionally, until the potatoes are very tender, about 10 minutes.

4. Remove from the heat and add about 2 cups of the vegetables to a blender or food processor. Puree until smooth, then add to the soup and return to the heat.

5. Add the milk and chopped clams and simmer for about 5 minutes to blend the flavors. Stir in the salt, pepper, and parsley. Garnish with the bacon (if desired).

Per serving *(1 cup): 126 calories, 3 g fat, 1 g saturated fat, 11 mg cholesterol, 138 mg sodium, 17 g carbohydrate, 2 g fiber, 8 g protein.*

▶ Lentil Soup with Root Vegetables

Makes 9 cups

2 cups brown lentils

1 tablespoon olive oil

1 large onion, diced

2 stalks celery, diced

2 cloves garlic, finely chopped

8 ounces turnip or parsnip, diced

2 large carrots, diced

2 quarts beef or vegetable stock

1 tablespoon tomato paste

¼ teaspoon dried thyme

1 bay leaf

⅛ teaspoon each salt and pepper

1. Rinse the lentils in a sieve under cold water. Pick them over, discarding any small stones.

2. Heat the oil in a 4-quart saucepan over medium heat. Add the onion, celery, and garlic and cook, stirring constantly, until softened and golden brown, about 6 minutes. Add the turnip and carrots, then about ¼ cup of the stock. Cook, stirring frequently, until slightly soft.

3. Add the lentils, tomato paste, thyme, bay leaf, and the remaining stock and stir to combine. Bring to a boil, then reduce the heat and partially cover. Simmer, stirring occasionally, until the lentils and vegetables are very tender, about 50 minutes. Add the salt and pepper. Remove and discard the bay leaf before serving.

Per serving *(1 cup): 217 calories, 3 g fat, 1 g saturated fat, 0 mg cholesterol, 160 mg sodium, 35 g carbohydrate, 8 g fiber, 15 g protein.*

▶ Grilled Corn Pasta Salad

Makes 8 servings

4 large ears sweet corn in husks

2 cups cooked medium tube pasta

2 cups cherry tomatoes

1 medium zucchini, thinly sliced

½ cup sliced black olives

⅓ cup vinegar

2 tablespoons olive or canola oil

1 tablespoon chopped fresh basil or 1 teaspoon dried basil

1 teaspoon sugar

1 teaspoon salt

½ teaspoon ground mustard

¼ teaspoon garlic powder

¼ teaspoon fresh-ground black pepper

1. Grill the corn in the husks over medium heat, covered and turning often, until tender, 10 to 15 minutes. Let cool and cut the corn off the cob.

2. In a large bowl, combine the corn, pasta, tomatoes, zucchini, and olives.

3. In a small bowl, combine the vinegar, oil, basil, sugar, salt, mustard, garlic powder, and pepper. Mix well. Pour over the vegetables and stir gently. Cover and refrigerate until ready to serve.

Per serving: *164 calories, 6 g fat, 1 g saturated fat, 0 mg cholesterol, 382 mg sodium, 27 g carbohydrate, 3 g fiber, 5 g protein.*

▶ Tuscan Bean Salad

Makes 4 servings

1 cup dried navy beans, sorted and rinsed

4 cups cold water

½ cup finely chopped red onion

½ cup thinly sliced celery

¼ cup chopped parsley

3 tablespoons chicken broth

2 tablespoons balsamic vinegar

1 tablespoon olive or canola oil

1 teaspoon Dijon mustard

½ teaspoon minced garlic

1 teaspoon salt

¼ teaspoon ground oregano

¼ teaspoon ground thyme

1. Place the beans in a Dutch oven or large saucepan and add water to cover by 2 inches. Bring to a boil. Boil for 2 minutes, then remove from the heat, cover, and let stand for 1 hour. Drain and rinse the beans, discarding the liquid.

2. Return the beans to the pan and add the cold water. Bring to a boil, then reduce the heat, cover, and simmer until tender, 50 to 60 minutes. Drain. In a large bowl, combine the beans, onion, celery, and parsley.

3. In a jar with a tight-fitting lid, combine the broth, vinegar, oil, mustard, garlic, salt, oregano, and thyme. Shake well, pour over the bean mixture, and stir to coat. Cover and refrigerate for at least 2 hours.

Per serving: *224 calories, 4 g fat, 1 g saturated fat, 0 mg cholesterol, 682 mg sodium, 36 g carbohydrate, 14 g fiber, 12 g protein.*

▶ New Waldorf Salad

Makes 4 servings

1 medium red apple, chopped

1 medium green apple, chopped

1 medium pear, chopped

½ cup green grapes

¼ cup raisins

¼ cup slivered almonds, toasted

1 carton (6 ounces) reduced-fat lemon yogurt

2 teaspoons lemon juice

2 teaspoons orange juice

2 teaspoons honey

1 teaspoon grated orange zest

Lettuce leaves *(optional)*

1. In a large bowl, combine the apples, pear, grapes, raisins, and almonds.

2. In a small bowl, combine the yogurt, lemon juice, orange juice, honey, and orange zest. Pour over the fruit and stir to coat. Serve immediately in lettuce-lined bowls (if desired).

Per serving: *193 calories, 5 g fat, 1 g saturated fat, 2 mg cholesterol, 33 mg sodium, 35 g carbohydrate, 4 g fiber, 5 g protein.*

▶ Spinach Salad with Honey Dressing

Makes 10 servings

1 bag (10 ounces) fresh spinach, trimmed, washed, and torn

1 small head iceberg lettuce, torn

2 scallions, thinly sliced

3 tablespoons chopped green bell pepper

1 medium cucumber, quartered and sliced

2 large oranges, cut into bite-size pieces

½ cup sunflower seeds

¾ cup fat-free mayonnaise

2 tablespoons honey

1 tablespoon lemon juice

1. In a large bowl, combine the spinach, lettuce, scallions, pepper, cucumber, oranges, and sunflower seeds.

2. In a small bowl, combine the mayonnaise, honey, and lemon juice and stir until smooth. Pour over the salad and toss to coat. Serve immediately.

Per serving: *100 calories, 4 g fat, 1 g saturated fat, 0 mg cholesterol, 100 mg sodium, 16 g carbohydrate, 4 g fiber, 3 g protein.*

▶ Cauliflower Provençal

Makes 4 servings

1 cauliflower
1 sweet red pepper, diced
2 tomatoes, coarsely chopped
⅓ cup vegetable stock
¼ cup sliced black olives
⅛ teaspoon each salt and pepper

1. Cut off leaves and stem of cauliflower. Break florets from core. Steam until just tender, about 9 minutes. In a saucepan, combine red pepper, tomatoes, and stock. Bring to a boil over moderate heat. Cover pan and cook, stirring, until peppers are almost tender, about 3 minutes.

2. Add cauliflower and olives and toss to coat. Cover pan and continue to cook, stirring, until cauliflower is tender, about 2 to 3 minutes. Season with salt and pepper.

Per serving: *74 calories, 1 g fat, 0 g saturated fat, 0 mg cholesterol, 127 mg sodium, 14 g carbohydrate, 1 g fiber, 5 g protein.*

▶ Corn Pudding

Makes 4 servings

½ teaspoon olive or canola oil
1 slice reduced-sodium bacon, coarsely chopped
2 leeks, trimmed and chopped
1 small sweet red pepper, finely chopped
2 cups corn kernels
2 cups cubed bread
¾ cup 1% low-fat milk
1 egg
1 egg white
¼ teaspoon dry mustard
⅛ teaspoon each salt and pepper

1. Lightly grease a 1½-quart baking dish or casserole with oil. Preheat oven to 350°F.

2. In a nonstick skillet, cook bacon over moderate heat until crisp and fat is rendered. Add leeks and sweet pepper and sauté until softened, about 3 to 4 minutes. Remove from the heat and pour into baking dish. Stir in corn and bread.

3. In a bowl, whisk milk, egg, egg white, mustard, salt, and pepper. Pour mixture into baking dish and stir to combine. Bake pudding until puffed and cooked through, about 30 to 40 minutes.

Per serving: *195 calories, 4 g fat, 1 g saturated fat, 56 mg cholesterol, 217 mg sodium, 35 g carbohydrate, 4 g fiber, 9 g protein.*

▶ Oven Fries

Makes 4 servings

2 pounds large baking potatoes or sweet potatoes, scrubbed but unpeeled
2 teaspoons olive or canola oil
⅛ teaspoon each salt and pepper

1. Place 2 baking sheets in the oven and preheat the oven to 450°F. Cut the potatoes lengthwise into ½-inch slices, then cut the slices lengthwise into ½-inch strips.

2. In a large bowl, combine the oil with the salt and pepper. Add the potatoes and toss well so that they are evenly coated. Arrange the potatoes in a single layer on the hot baking sheets and bake, turning once, until browned, crisp, and cooked through, about 30 to 35 minutes.

Per serving: *150 calories, 2 g fat, 0 g saturated fat, 0 mg cholesterol, 72 mg sodium, 29 g carbohydrate, 3 g fiber, 4 g protein.*

▶ Skillet Vegetable Side Dish

Makes 8 servings

3   carrots, thinly sliced
1   large onion, chopped
1/2 medium head cabbage, chopped
1/2 medium green bell pepper, chopped
1   tablespoon chopped celery
2   cloves garlic, minced
2   tablespoons Worcester-shire sauce
1   tablespoon minced parsley
1   teaspoon caraway seeds
1   teaspoon Italian seasoning

Coat a large skillet with cooking spray. Add the carrots, onion, cabbage, pepper, and celery and stir-fry over medium-high heat for 5 minutes. Add the garlic, Worcestershire sauce, parsley, caraway seeds, and seasoning. Stir-fry until the vegetables are cooked to desired doneness, about 5 minutes.

Per serving: *50 calories, 1 g fat, 0 g saturated fat, 0 mg cholesterol, 50 mg sodium, 13 g carbohydrate, 3 g fiber, 2 g protein.*

▶ Ginger-Orange Squash

Makes 4 servings

1   butternut squash (2 pounds)
2   tablespoons frozen orange juice concentrate
2   tablespoons brown sugar
2   teaspoons margarine
1/4 teaspoon ground ginger

1. Place the squash on a microwavable plate and pierce several times with a knife or fork. Microwave on high for 5 minutes. Slice into quarters and remove the seeds. Return to the plate cut side down, cover with wax paper, and microwave for 7 minutes. Turn and microwave until soft, 6 to 8 minutes.

2. Scoop out the pulp. In a medium bowl, combine the pulp, juice concentrate, brown sugar, margarine, and ginger.

Per serving: *150 calories, 2 g fat, 1 g saturated fat, 0 mg cholesterol, 10 mg sodium, 34 g carbohydrate, 5 g fiber, 2 g protein.*

▶ Fish Baked on a Bed of Broccoli, Corn, and Red Pepper

Makes 4 servings

4 sole or any firm white fillets (4–6 ounces each), fresh or frozen and thawed

2 tablespoons fat-free Italian dressing or vinaigrette

1 tablespoon fine dry unseasoned bread crumbs

1 tablespoon grated Parmesan cheese

¼ teaspoon paprika

1 tablespoon olive or canola oil

2 cups broccoli florets

1 cup fresh or frozen corn kernels, thawed

1 sweet red pepper, cut into thin strips

1 small red onion, thinly sliced

2 tablespoons chopped parsley or 2 teaspoons dried

1 tablespoon chopped fresh basil or 1 teaspoon dried

⅛ teaspoon each salt and pepper

1. Place the fish in a shallow baking dish and brush lightly with the Italian dressing. Cover and refrigerate.

2. In a small bowl, combine the bread crumbs with the Parmesan cheese and paprika until blended. Preheat the oven to 425°F. Brush 4 individual dishes or one 13 x 9 x 2-inch ovenproof dish with oil.

3. In a large bowl, combine the broccoli, corn, red pepper, onion, parsley, basil, salt, and pepper. Divide the vegetable mixture evenly among the dishes. Cover with aluminum foil and bake until the vegetables are just tender, 35 to 40 minutes.

4. Uncover the dishes and top vegetables with fish fillets. Cover again and bake until fish is barely cooked and still moist in thickest part, about 8 to 10 minutes.

5. Uncover the dishes, sprinkle with the bread crumb mixture, and continue to bake, uncovered, until the topping is golden, about 2 to 3 minutes longer.

Per serving: 210 calories, 6 g fat, 1 g saturated fat, 56 mg cholesterol, 340 mg sodium, 16 g carbohydrate, 3 g fiber, 25 g protein.

▶ Shrimp Jambalaya

Makes 4 servings

2 slices reduced-sodium bacon

1 ounce turkey sausage, sliced

1 large onion, diced

2 cloves garlic, finely chopped

1 sweet green pepper, diced

2 stalks celery, diced

1¾ cups chicken stock

1 can (14 ounces) reduced-sodium tomatoes

¼ cup chopped parsley

1 box (7 ounces) wild pecan rice or 1 cup long-grain rice

½ teaspoon hot red pepper sauce

½ teaspoon dried thyme

1 bay leaf

¼ teaspoon pepper

12 ounces medium shrimp, peeled and deveined

1. In a 4-quart saucepan, cook the bacon over moderate heat until crisp. Using a slotted spoon, transfer bacon to a plate.

2. Add the sausage slices to the pan and cook, stirring frequently, until browned, about 5 minutes. Transfer to the plate with the bacon.

3. Add onion, garlic, green pepper, and celery and sauté, stirring, about 5 minutes. If necessary, add a little stock to keep vegetables from browning.

4. Stir the tomatoes, remaining stock, parsley, rice, hot red pepper sauce, thyme, bay leaf, and pepper into the vegetables. Bring the mixture to a boil. Cover pan and simmer until rice is just tender and most of the liquid has been absorbed, about 20 to 30 minutes.

5. Stir in shrimp, sausage, and bacon. Cover and continue to simmer until shrimp are pink and firm, about 5 minutes longer. Discard bay leaf.

Per serving: *376 calories, 8 g fat, 3 g saturated fat, 113 mg cholesterol, 316 mg sodium, 54 g carbohydrate, 4 g fiber, 22 g protein.*

▶ Lemony Salmon Patties

Makes 4 servings

Salmon Patties

- 1 can (14³/₄ ounces) pink salmon, drained, skin and bones removed
- ³/₄ cup fat-free milk
- 1 cup soft bread crumbs
- 1 egg, beaten
- 1 tablespoon chopped parsley
- 1 teaspoon minced onion
- ¹/₂ teaspoon Worcestershire sauce
- ¹/₈ teaspoon pepper

Lemon Sauce

- ³/₄ cup fat-free milk
- 4 teaspoons all-purpose flour
- 2 tablespoons lemon juice
- ¹/₄ teaspoon cayenne pepper

1. Preheat the oven to 350°F. Coat an 8-cup muffin pan with cooking spray.

2. *To make the salmon patties:* In a large bowl, combine the salmon, milk, bread crumbs, egg, parsley, onion, Worcestershire sauce, and pepper. Mix well. Spoon ¹/₄ cup of the mixture into each muffin cup. Bake until browned, about 45 minutes.

3. *To make the lemon sauce:* In a small saucepan over medium heat, gradually stir the milk into the flour. Bring to a boil, stirring constantly, and cook until thickened, about 2 minutes. Remove from the heat and stir in the lemon juice and cayenne. Serve over patties.

Per serving: *220 calories, 6 g fat, 1 g saturated fat, 130 mg cholesterol, 470 mg sodium, 13 g carbohydrate, 0 g fiber, 32 g protein.*

▶ Mediterranean Baked Fish

Makes 4 servings

- 1 cup thinly sliced leeks (white parts only)
- 2 cloves garlic, minced
- 2 teaspoons olive or canola oil
- 12 large leaves basil
- 1¹/₂ pounds orange roughy fillets
- 1 teaspoon salt
- 2 plum tomatoes, sliced
- 1 can (2¹/₂ ounces) sliced black olives, drained
- 1 medium lemon
- ¹/₈ teaspoon fresh-ground black pepper
- 4 sprigs rosemary

1. Preheat the oven to 425°F. Coat a 13 x 9 x 2-inch baking dish with cooking spray.

2. In a medium nonstick skillet, sauté the leeks and garlic in the oil until tender; set aside. Arrange the basil in a single layer in the baking dish and top with the fish. Sprinkle with the salt and top with the leek mixture. Arrange the tomatoes and olives over the fish.

3. Thinly slice half of the lemon and place on top of the fish. Squeeze the juice from the remaining lemon half over all. Sprinkle with the pepper. Cover and bake until the fish flakes easily with a fork, 15 to 20 minutes. Garnish with the rosemary.

Per serving: *186 calories, 6 g fat, 1 g saturated fat, 34 mg cholesterol, 857 mg sodium, 9 g carbohydrate, 3 g fiber, 26 g protein.*

▶ Zesty Apricot Turkey

Makes 4 servings

- 1/3 cup reduced-sugar apricot preserves
- 1 tablespoon white-wine or cider vinegar
- 1 tablespoon honey
- 1/2 teaspoon grated lemon zest
- 1 clove garlic, minced
- 1/8 teaspoon hot red pepper sauce
- 1 boneless skinless turkey breast half (1 pound)

1. In a microwavable bowl, combine the preserves, vinegar, honey, lemon zest, garlic, and red pepper sauce. Microwave, uncovered, on high until the preserves melt, 1 to 2 minutes. Stir to blend. Set aside half to serve with the turkey.

2. Grill the turkey, covered, over indirect medium heat for 3 minutes on each side. Brush with the remaining apricot sauce and grill until the juices run clear and a meat thermometer reads 170°F, 7 to 10 minutes. Slice and serve with the reserved sauce.

Per serving: *193 calories, 1 g fat, 0 g saturated fat, 70 mg cholesterol, 62 mg sodium, 17 g carbohydrate, 1 g fiber, 28 g protein.*

▶ Lemon Chicken Tacos

Makes 4 servings

- 1 pound boneless skinless chicken breasts, cut into 1/2-inch cubes
- 2 tablespoons plus 1 teaspoon lemon juice
- 1 large onion, sliced
- 1 green onion, sliced
- 2 cloves garlic, minced
- 2 teaspoons olive or canola oil
- 1/2 teaspoon ground cumin
- 1/2 teaspoon salt
- 1/4 teaspoon fresh-ground black pepper
- 2 plum tomatoes, seeded and chopped
- 1/4 cup minced cilantro or parsley
- 8 flour tortillas (8 inches), warmed
- 1 cup shredded lettuce
- 1/2 cup salsa

1. Place the chicken in a large zip-close plastic bag and add 2 tablespoons of the lemon juice. Seal the bag and turn to coat. Refrigerate for 1 to 2 hours.

2. In a large nonstick skillet, sauté the onions and garlic in the oil until tender. Add the chicken, cumin, salt, and pepper and cook, stirring, until the juices run clear, 4 minutes. Remove from the heat and stir in the tomatoes, cilantro, and the remaining lemon juice. Spoon onto the tortillas and top with lettuce. Serve with the salsa.

Per serving: *(2 tacos): 371 calories, 6 g fat, 1 g saturated fat, 66 mg cholesterol, 599 mg sodium, 44 g carbohydrate, 4 g fiber, 36 g protein.*

▶ Herbed Lime Chicken

Makes 4 servings

1 bottle (16 ounces) fat-free Italian salad dressing

½ cup lime juice

1 lime, halved and sliced

3 cloves garlic, minced

1 teaspoon dried thyme

4 boneless skinless chicken breast halves (1 pound)

1. In a medium bowl, combine the salad dressing, lime juice, lime, garlic, and thyme. Remove ½ cup for basting; cover and refrigerate. Pour the remaining marinade into a large zip-close plastic bag and add the chicken. Seal the bag and turn to coat. Refrigerate for 8 to 10 hours.

2. Drain and discard the marinade. Grill the chicken, uncovered, over medium heat for 5 minutes. Turn and baste with the reserved marinade. Grill, basting occasionally, until the juices run clear, 5 to 7 minutes.

Per serving: 162 calories, 2 g fat, 1 g saturated fat, 67 mg cholesterol, 718 mg sodium, 8 g carbohydrate, 0 g fiber, 27 g protein.

▶ Cranberry Chicken

Makes 6 servings

½ cup all-purpose flour

¼ teaspoon fresh-ground black pepper

6 boneless skinless chicken breast halves (1½ pounds)

3 tablespoons margarine

1 cup water

1 cup fresh or frozen cranberries

½ cup packed brown sugar

Dash ground nutmeg

1 tablespoon red-wine vinegar *(optional)*

Hot cooked rice *(optional)*

1. In a shallow dish, combine the flour and pepper and dredge the chicken.

2. Melt the margarine in a large skillet over medium heat. Add the chicken and brown on both sides. Remove from the skillet and keep warm.

3. Add the water, cranberries, brown sugar, nutmeg, and vinegar (if desired) to the skillet. Cook, stirring, until the berries burst, about 5 minutes. Return the chicken to the skillet. Cover and simmer, basting occasionally with the sauce, until tender, 20 to 30 minutes. Serve over the rice (if desired).

Per serving (calculated without vinegar and rice): 290 calories, 7 g fat, 2 g saturated fat, 65 mg cholesterol, 80 mg sodium, 28 g carbohydrate, 1 g fiber, 27 g protein

▶ Spinach-Stuffed Meat Loaf

Makes 6 servings

1 pound lean ground beef

8 ounces lean ground turkey

1 small onion, finely chopped

½ cup fresh bread crumbs

⅛ teaspoon garlic salt

1 tablespoon tomato paste

1 egg white

½ cup part-skim ricotta cheese

1 package (10 ounces) frozen chopped spinach, thawed and drained

⅛ teaspoon each salt and pepper

2 large onions, thinly sliced

2 carrots, coarsely chopped

1 can (28 ounces) crushed tomatoes

1. In a bowl, mix beef, turkey, chopped onion, bread crumbs, garlic salt, and tomato paste. In another bowl, mix egg white, ricotta, spinach, salt, and pepper. Preheat oven to 350°F.

2. Turn out the beef mixture onto a large sheet of wax paper, and form into a 9- by 10-inch rectangle with your hands. Spoon the spinach stuffing lengthwise down the center of the meat, leaving about 1 inch uncovered at each short end.

3. With the help of the wax paper, lift the long edges of the meat. Fold the meat over the stuffing to enclose it. Using your fingers, pinch the edges of the meat together.

4. Place loaf seam side down in a nonstick roasting pan. Add onions, carrots, and tomatoes to pan.

5. Bake until meat and vegetables are cooked, about 1½ hours. Transfer meat to platter. Puree vegetables in a blender and serve sauce with the meat loaf.

Per serving: *294 calories, 6 g fat, 2 g saturated fat, 71 mg cholesterol, 405 mg sodium, 28 g carbohydrate, 2 g fiber, 32 g protein.*

▶ Beef and Turkey Chili

Makes 6 servings

1 pound lean ground beef

8 ounces lean ground turkey

1 tablespoon olive or canola oil

2 large onions, coarsely chopped

3 cloves garlic, finely chopped

3 sweet red or green peppers, coarsely chopped

1 tablespoon chili powder or more to taste

1 teaspoon each ground cumin and coriander

1 can (28 ounces) crushed tomatoes

Dash of hot red pepper sauce *(optional)*

1/8 teaspoon pepper

1 package (10 ounces) frozen corn kernels, thawed

1 can (16 ounces) red kidney beans, drained and rinsed

1. Heat a Dutch oven over moderately high heat until hot. Add the beef and turkey and sauté, stirring frequently, until the meat has lost its pink color and has released its juices, about 7 minutes.

2. Remove from the heat and spoon the meat into a sieve set over a bowl. Allow all the fat to drain from the meat; it will take at least 10 minutes.

3. Meanwhile, in the Dutch oven, heat the oil over moderate heat. Add the onions and garlic and sauté until softened and golden brown, about 5 to 7 minutes. Stir in the sweet peppers, chili powder, and spices and cook until the peppers are slightly soft, about 5 minutes longer. Return the meat to the pan.

4. Stir in the crushed tomatoes, hot red pepper sauce, if using, and pepper and bring to a boil. Partially cover and simmer, stirring occasionally, until the sauce thickens, about 20 to 30 minutes.

5. Stir in the corn kernels and kidney beans. Cover and cook about 5 minutes longer to heat through.

Per serving: *340 calories, 7 g fat, 2 g saturated fat, 68 mg cholesterol, 546 mg sodium, 37 g carbohydrate, 8 g fiber, 34 g protein.*

▶ Spicy Beef and Turkey Tacos

Makes 8 servings

1	pound lean ground beef
8	ounces lean ground turkey
1	tablespoon olive or canola oil
1	onion, coarsely chopped
3	cloves garlic
1	red or green bell pepper
1	tablespoon chili powder, or more to taste
1	can (16 ounces) crushed tomatoes, drained
1/8	teaspoon each salt and pepper
16	taco shells
3	cups shredded iceberg lettuce
1/2	cup shredded jalapeño cheese or low-fat cheddar cheese

1. Heat a Dutch oven over medium-high heat. Add beef and turkey; cook, stirring frequently, until meat is no longer pink and releases its juices, about 7 minutes. Remove from heat and drain in a sieve set over a bowl; at least 10 minutes.

2. Meanwhile, heat the oil in the Dutch oven over medium heat. Add the onion and finely chopped garlic and cook until softened and golden brown, 5 to 7 minutes. Stir in the bell pepper, coarsely chopped, and chili powder and cook until the pepper is slightly soft, about 5 minutes. Return the meat to the pan.

3. Preheat the oven according to the taco shell package directions. Stir the tomatoes, salt, and pepper into the pan and bring to a boil. Cover and simmer, stirring occasionally, until the mixture resembles a rich stew, about 15 minutes.

4. On a baking sheet, warm the taco shells according to the package directions. Divide the meat mixture among the shells, then sprinkle with the lettuce and cheese.

Per serving: *293 calories, 12 g fat, 3 g saturated fat, 61 mg cholesterol, 257 mg sodium, 21 g carbohydrate, 3 g fiber, 26 g protein.*

▶ Sweet-and-Sour Pork

Makes 6 servings

2 teaspoons vegetable oil

1 pound boneless lean pork, cut into 1-inch cubes

1 teaspoon paprika

⅓ cup water

3 tablespoons brown sugar

2 tablespoons cornstarch

1 can (20 ounces) unsweetened pineapple chunks, drained and juice reserved

⅓ cup vinegar

1 tablespoon soy sauce

1 teaspoon Worcester-shire sauce

1 green bell pepper, sliced

1 small onion, sliced

1 can (8 ounces) sliced water chestnuts, drained

Hot cooked rice *(optional)*

1. Heat the oil in a wok or skillet over medium-high heat. Add the pork, sprinkle with the paprika, and brown on all sides. Reduce the heat and add the water. Cover and simmer until tender, 20 to 25 minutes.

2. Meanwhile, in a medium bowl, combine the brown sugar and cornstarch. Gradually add the reserved pineapple juice, vinegar, soy sauce, and Worcestershire sauce and stir until smooth. Add to the pork, increase the heat to medium, and cook, stirring constantly, until thick and bubbly. Cook, stirring, for 2 minutes longer.

3. Stir in the pineapple, pepper, onion, and water chestnuts. Cover and simmer until the vegetables are crisp-tender, 5 minutes. Serve over the rice (if desired).

Per serving *(calculated without rice): 290 calories, 9 g fat, 3 g saturated fat, 65 mg cholesterol, 140 mg sodium, 28 g carbohydrate, 4 g fiber, 23 g protein.*

▶ Citrus-Topped Pork Chops

Makes 6 servings

6 loin pork chops (1 inch thick), trimmed

Fresh-ground black pepper to taste

¼ teaspoon paprika

½ cup apple jelly

1 cup orange juice

½ teaspoon lemon juice

1 teaspoon ground mustard

Dash ground ginger

6 slices orange

6 slices lemon

1. Coat a large skillet with cooking spray. Add the pork and brown on both sides over medium-high heat. Season with the pepper and paprika.

2. In a small bowl, combine the jelly, orange juice, lemon juice, mustard, and ginger. Pour over the pork, cover, and simmer for 15 minutes. Turn the pork, cover, and simmer for 15 minutes. Top each chop with an orange slice and a lemon slice. Cover and cook until the juices run clear, 6 to 8 minutes.

Per serving: *190 calories, 7 g fat, 3 g saturated fat, 53 mg cholesterol, 60 mg sodium, 26 g carbohydrate, 1 g fiber, 16 g protein.*

▶ Pork Loin Stuffed with Winter Fruits *Makes 6 servings*

¾ cup chicken stock

1 cup pitted prunes, coarsely chopped

1 cup dried apricots, coarsely chopped

2 pounds boneless pork loin

⅛ teaspoon salt

⅛ teaspoon fresh-ground black pepper

1 clove garlic, finely chopped

1 teaspoon dried thyme

2 tablespoons Madeira or port wine *(optional)*

2 tablespoons dark molasses

1. Bring the stock to a boil in a small saucepan over medium heat. Remove from the heat and stir in the prunes and apricots. Set aside to soak until very soft, at least 15 minutes.

2. Meanwhile, preheat the oven to 325°F. With a sharp knife, trim all the fat from the pork. Open the loin and pat dry with paper towels. Season the inside with the salt and pepper.

3. Drain the fruit, reserving the liquid in a saucepan. Spread the fruit on one of the long sides of the pork and scatter the garlic and thyme on top.

4. Fold the long edge of the pork over the fruit and roll up. With kitchen string, tie the roll at regular intervals to seal in the stuffing. Trim off the excess string. Place the pork on a rack in a roasting pan, seam side down, and bake for about 30 minutes.

5. Meanwhile, add the wine (if desired) and molasses to the reserved soaking liquid to make glaze, and bring to a boil.

6. Brush the glaze evenly over the pork. Bake, brushing with the glaze every 10 minutes, until tender and a meat thermometer inserted in the center of the pork reads 170°F, about 1 hour.

Per serving: *375 calories, 11 g fat, 4 g saturated fat, 95 mg cholesterol, 170 mg sodium, 34 g carbohydrate, 4 g fiber, 35 g protein.*

▶ Harvest Snack Cake

Makes 15 servings

2 cups whole wheat flour
1¼ cups packed brown sugar
2 teaspoons baking soda
¾ teaspoon ground cinnamon
½ teaspoon ground nutmeg
⅛ teaspoon ground ginger
2 eggs
½ cup unsweetened applesauce
1 teaspoon vanilla extract
1½ cups shredded carrots
1 cup raisins

1. Preheat the oven to 350°F. Coat a 13 x 9 x 2-inch baking pan with cooking spray.

2. In a large bowl, combine the flour, brown sugar, baking soda, cinnamon, nutmeg, and ginger. In a small bowl, combine the eggs, applesauce, and vanilla. Stir into the dry ingredients just until moistened.

3. With a rubber spatula, fold in the carrots and raisins (the batter will be thick), then spread evenly in the baking pan. Bake until a toothpick inserted near the center comes out clean, 30 to 35 minutes. Cool on a wire rack.

Per serving: 170 calories, 1 g fat, 0 g saturated fat, 28 mg cholesterol, 191 mg sodium, 39 g carbohydrate, 3 g fiber, 3 g protein.

▶ Walnut-Raisin Pudding

Makes 4 servings

½ cup orange juice
1 egg yolk
1 teaspoon honey
1 teaspoon vanilla extract
⅔ cup cooked rice
¼ cup raisins
¼ cup chopped walnuts, toasted
3 egg whites
Vegetable oil cooking spray

1. Preheat oven to 325°F. In a large mixing bowl, mix the orange juice with the egg yolk, honey, and vanilla extract.

2. Stir in the cooked rice, raisins, and toasted walnuts. In another bowl, whip the egg whites until soft peaks form, then carefully fold into the mixture with a large metal spoon.

3. Pour into 4 custard dishes that have been lightly coated with vegetable oil spray or lightly greased with vegetable oil.

4. Place custard dishes in a 13 x 9 x 2-inch baking pan and carefully add boiling water to the baking pan to a depth of 1 inch. Bake, uncovered, until just set, 30 to 35 minutes.

Per serving: 162 calories, 5 g fat, 3 g saturated fat, 53 mg cholesterol, 46 mg sodium, 24 g carbohydrate, 1 g fiber, 6 g protein.

▶ Apricot and Pear Compote

Makes 4 servings

1⅓ cups orange juice
     Finely grated zest and
     juice of 1 lemon
2   tablespoons honey
2   teaspoons vanilla
     extract
1   clove
8   fresh apricots, halved
2   firm but ripe pears,
     quartered
2   tablespoons raisins

1. In a saucepan, combine orange juice, lemon zest and juice, honey, vanilla extract, and clove. Bring to a boil, then reduce heat and simmer for 5 minutes.

2. Add the apricots and pears and bring to a boil. Reduce the heat, cover, and simmer until the fruit is just tender, 5 to 8 minutes.

3. Add the raisins, then remove the pan from the heat and allow to cool to room temperature in the syrup. Remove the clove before serving.

Per serving: 171 calories, 1 g fat, 0 g saturated fat, 0 mg cholesterol, 3 mg sodium, 43 g carbohydrate, 4 g fiber, 2 g protein.

▶ Peach Cobbler

Makes 6 servings

¼   cup peach nectar or
     water
¼   cup peach or apricot
     preserves
1   tablespoon cornstarch
1   teaspoon lemon juice
2   cups frozen peaches,
     thawed and cubed

Topping

⅓   cup whole wheat flour
⅓   cup all-purpose flour
¼   cup rolled oats
2   tablespoons brown
     sugar
1   teaspoon baking powder
¼   teaspoon ground
     cinnamon
1   egg
¼   cup 1% low-fat milk

1. Lightly grease an 8 x 8 x 2-inch baking dish. In a medium saucepan, combine the peach nectar, preserves, cornstarch, and lemon juice and stir until blended.

2. Stir in the peaches and cook over moderate heat for about 5 minutes, stirring constantly, until the mixture boils and thickens. Boil for 1 minute, stirring constantly. Remove from the heat and cover to keep warm. Preheat oven to 400°F.

3. *To make the topping:* In a medium mixing bowl, combine the flours, oats, brown sugar, baking powder, and cinnamon. Mix the egg and milk together in a cup and add to the flour mixture. Mix to form a soft, spoonable dough. Transfer the peach mixture to the baking dish.

4. Using a spoon, drop small portions of the dough over the peaches to make a "cobbled" effect. Bake until bubbling, crisp, and golden, 20 to 30 minutes.

Per serving: 190 calories, 1 g fat, 0 g saturated fat, 36 mg cholesterol, 71 mg sodium, 42 g carbohydrate, 3 g fiber, 4 g protein.

▶ Raspberry Dessert Sauce with Cantaloupe

Makes 4 servings

1 package (12 ounces) frozen raspberries
1 teaspoon lemon juice
2 tablespoons honey
1 medium cantaloupe
Fresh mint leaves

1. Reserve a few raspberries for garnish and keep them frozen. In a food processor or blender, puree the remaining raspberries until smooth. Strain the puree through a medium-fine sieve.

2. Add fresh lemon juice and honey to the raspberry puree and stir to mix well. Set aside.

3. Cut the cantaloupe into quarters and remove the seeds and rind. Using a sharp knife, slice each quarter lengthwise without cutting completely through. Open out each quarter into a fan shape.

4. Spread a quarter of the raspberry puree on the center of four 10-inch plates. Place a cantaloupe fan on each plate and decorate with fresh mint leaves and the reserved raspberries.

Per serving: 135 calories, 1 g fat, 0 g saturated fat, 0 mg cholesterol, 16 mg sodium, 33 g carbohydrate, 7 g fiber, 2 g protein.

Index

133, 151–52, 179

monitoring, 27–28, 60, 210

Blood sugar metabolism, improving, 104, 132. *See also* Insulin resistance; Metabolic syndrome

BMI. *See* Body mass index

Body fat, 20–22. *See also* Visceral fat

Body mass index (BMI), 21

walking and, 138

Bread, 69, 83, 117

Breakfast, 116

high-fiber, 68–69

recipes

Apple-Topped Oatcakes, 226

Hearty Carrot Muffins, 227

Hearty Ham Scramble, 225

Oatmeal Waffles, 225

Potatoes O'Brien, 227

Smoothie, 70

Vegetable Omelet, 70

restaurant, 119

sample meals for, 70

for weight loss, 77

Breathing

deep, 179, 195

in strength training, 150

Broccoli, 100

Buddy system, for exercise motivation, 54, 143

Bulgur, 69

Bupropion (Zyban), 195

Butter, in restaurant food, 118

B vitamins, 44, 101, 121, 128. *See also* Niacin

C

Calcium, 69, 97, 102, 128

Calorie(s), 76–77

burning, with activity, 147

needs, daily, 76–77, 208–9

Canola oil, 66, 110, 114

Carbohydrates, 88–92. *See also* Low-carbohydrate diets

complex, 90, 92

glycemic index of, 89

net (smart or impact), 90

simple (refined), 22, 83–84, 90, 91–92

whole grains, 68–69

Carbon monoxide from smoking, 192

Cardiovascular disease. *See* Heart disease

Cardiovascular fitness, 151

Carrots, 100

Heart Carrot Muffins, 227

Cast-iron skillet, iron from, 114

Cauliflower Provençal, 232

Causes of heart disease, 12. *See also* Heart attackers

Cereal, high fiber, 68–69, 92, 110

Cheese, for snacks, 71

Chest pain, as heart attack symptom, 12

Chewing tobacco, 194

Chicken, 64

Chicken Salad Wrap, 71–72

Cranberry Chicken, 238

Herbed Lime Chicken, 238

Lemon Chicken Tacos, 237

Chinese food, 116, 119

Chocolate, dark, 99

Cholesterol, 23–26

HDL (*see* HDL cholesterol)

heart disease risk and, 13

high blood pressure with high levels of, 19

LDL (*see* LDL cholesterol)

lowering with

foods, 97, 98, 99, 104

exercise, 133

fiber, 124

phytosterols, 125

statin drugs, 26, 282

testing, 60

Cigarettes. *See* Smoking

Cinnamon, 72, 104

Cinnamon Baked Apple, 75

Cinnamon Popcorn, 224

Citrus–Topped Pork Chops, 243

Cleaning, as exercise, 146

Clopidogrel (Plavix), 128

Clots, aspirin preventing, 128

Cocoa, 74, 99, 102

Coenzyme Q$_{10}$, 40, 126

Contraceptives, 14

Contract to quit smoking, 193

Greeks, heart health in, 11

Green tea, 75, 109

Grilled Corn Pasta Salad, 230

Gum disease, 33, 190, 199–200

H

Ham Scramble, Hearty, 225

Hand washing, for preventing infection, 190, 203, 204

Happiness, 17, 47, 168, 172, 173–75
  quiz for evaluating, 51

Harvest Snack Cake, 244

Hawthorn berry extract, 126

HDL cholesterol
  in cholesterol balance, 24
  effect of trans fats on, 82
  function of, 25, 39
  heart disease risk and, 13–14, 26
  monounsaturated fat increasing, 66
  niacin increasing, 128
  tracking, 210

Healthy Heart Starter Kit, 220–21

Heart
  damage, repairing, 126
  oxygen-deprived, 12
  role of, in blood pressure, 28

Heart attackers, 18–42
  apo(a) and apo(b), 42
  body fat, excess, 20–22
  cholesterol, 23–26
  chronic inflammation,

31–34
  high blood pressure, 27–30
  homocysteine, 41
  Lp(a), 41–42
  metabolic syndrome, 35–57
  nitric oxide deficiency, 42
  oxidative stress, 38–40
  triglycerides, 13–14, 25, 26

Heart attacks
  aspirin and, 127
  causes of, 12, 14–15 (see also Heart attackers)
  heart failure after, 11
  influenza and, 201
  LDL-ox and, 39
  metabolic syndrome and, 37
  refined grains and, 84
  second, 11
  symptoms of, 12, 13

Heartbeat irregularities, preventing, 123, 126

Heart disease
  in Americans, 11–12
  in animals, 15
  causes of, 12, 14–15 (see also Heart attackers)
  drawbacks of research on, 18
  risk factors, interwoven, 18–19 (see also Heart attackers)
  in women, 12–14
  worldwide death rates from, 10

Heart failure, 11, 12

Heart infection, preventing, 204

Heart rate, 13
  exercise lowering, 133, 151–52
  maximum, 148
  monitors, 148
  tracking, 211

Hearty Carrot Muffins, 227

Hearty Ham Scramble, 225

Helping others, 170–71

Herbal-enhanced foods, 80

Herbed Lime Chicken, 238

High blood pressure, 27–30, 210. See also Blood pressure
  contributors to, 84, 85, 177
  high cholesterol with, 19
  lowering, 30, 69, 98, 102, 104, 126, 127, 132, 133, 151–52, 179
  in women, 14

High cholesterol. See Cholesterol

High-fructose corn syrup, 86–87

Homemade Peach Soft-Serve, 75

Homocysteine, 41
  B vitamins to lower, 41, 121
  foods to lower, 92, 98, 100, 101, 103

Hormone replacement therapy (HRT), 14

Hormones
  blood pressure and, 28
  chronic inflammation and, 33

Hostility, 17, 172–73